Activate the Female Orgasm System

The Story of O-Shot ®

By **Charles Runels, MD**
Inventor of the O-Shot ® Procedure

Find more help at: www.OShot.info

Table of Contents

Introduction: Who I Am & Why I Wrote This Book

Hello,

How does anyone get the idea to draw blood from a woman's body and then inject it into her vagina (the O-Shot ® procedure)?

I'm **Charles Runels, the inventor of the O-Shot ® procedure, the first person in the world to use blood-derived growth factors to rejuvenate the vagina to improve sex and to stop urinary incontinence.**

I don't expect to ever think of anything that I will consider more important than the O-Shot ® procedure.

As you will see later in this book, **a woman helped me think of the idea (not a woman physician...a woman lover).** Since then, amazing physicians around the world have adopted the procedure and continue to work to improve the results of the method.

Yesterday, I received an email from a woman who wants to have coffee with me and personally thank me. She's 65-years-young and, after the O-Shot ® procedure, she's enjoying orgasms *for the first time in her life*. One of the nurse practitioners that I trained did her procedure. The patient wants to thank me because her relationship and *her life changed after the nurse practitioner gave her the O-Shot ®.*

Think about it...a woman, aged 65, whom I never met, now enjoys a better connection and more pleasure with her husband, and a changed life because of a 10-minute, pain-free procedure that is nearly risk free.

That pleases me very much.

Sometimes, I just sit and think of the thousands of people now, and I do mean right now in this present moment, who are enjoying amazing sex. Many of these people had given up on sex, feeling rejected and unlovable—until the O-Shot ® gave them back their sex lives.

That makes me smile.

Because of social repercussions, physicians largely ignored research into women's sexual problems (as compared to research about men's sexual problems, an open area of medicine). I tried to change that with the O-Shot ® procedure.

Because of those social repercussions, the following confessions were needed before I could think up the O-Shot ® procedure:

5 Critical Confessions of a Sex Doctor...

1. I am a man—a **psychological gender** (though some women tell me that I'm a homosexual woman stuck in a man's body).

2. I have a penis—a **physical gender.**

3. I **enjoy sex**—enjoying both my physical and psychological gender.

4. I like for other people to enjoy sex partly because I think *good sex helps build strong families* and partly because sex can be fun and even inspirational.

5. Medical doctors should help people find healthier and more enjoyable sex by improving the health of the *Orgasm System*.

Those may seem like obvious confessions. But for many reasons, **most physicians seem to struggle to admit or to discuss such things...and the research proves it!** Research shows that only 14% of women ever have a conversation about sex with their doctors even though 40% of women suffer distress due to sexual dysfunction. This low percentage of women who do ask their doctors about sex must do so largely because physicians avoid the subject.

Education is critical to good sex and I always encourage women to seek the counsel of a good sex educator (I've talked with many). But, it does no good to understand how to drive a car with a broken engine. Physicians must be willing--even eager--to do their part to keep the health of the body optimal for good sex else both the work of the educator and the romance of the lover becomes less effective.

In this book, I tell you how my desire for better sex for others and for myself led to the development of the O-Shot ® procedure.

In that story you will better understand the components of the Female Orgasm System as well as how to activate that system.

Dis-ease Leads to Extreme Pleasure

Around 1 out of 10 women never enjoy an orgasm in their entire life. Around 5 of 10 women of every age suffer with pain with sexual intercourse, or decreased desire, or inability to experience orgasm.

Around 4 out of 10 women have sexual dysfunction to the point that it's a serious psychological distress for them.

Also, around 1 out of 20 women in their 20's suffer with urinary incontinence severe enough to cause a hygiene or a social problem. The percentage goes up to nearly ½ of women by the time they reach 60.

The amazing benefit that evolved from seeking a treatment for sex problems is that the same treatment that takes women from dis-ease to healing (the O-Shot ® procedure) will also take a woman of normal functioning to a place of AMAZING sexual response.

These are not insignificant problems, and sex is not just about pleasure. Sex & beauty are the "scaffolding of love" according to Emerson.

Skyscrapers in New York City stand without scaffolding, but it would have been impossible to build them without scaffolding.

People mature in their relationship. Sex can become less important as we all become like the *Velveteen Rabbit*; but sex can be needed to establish relationships and continue to be of help in maintaining even the most mature relationship--which **carries over to maintaining families and happiness by the energy and the creativity and the comfort that results**.

So this book is not just about having fun; it's about happiness, creativity, prayer, and family. But, if we could make sex more fun, would that be a bad thing?

Use Sex to Increase Creativity

Throughout time, philosophers and poets have written that sex—if practiced correctly—gives energy, increases one's creativity and inventiveness, leading to better financial situations and even to more connection during prayer. Over the past twenty plus years as a physician, I have treated thousands of people who have healthy sex drives and are channeled in the right direction. These people make more money, they have more friends, and they enjoy stronger families. Meanwhile, those who suffer with sex problems may still flourish, but life can be more difficult.

When **Sigmund Freud talked about Leonardo da Vinci** gaining much of his creativity by the way he channeled his sexual energy, the research for the O-Shot ® was justified—sexual energy fuels genius.

When **Benjamin Franklin** wrote in his autobiography about his sexual practices and how those practices led to his productivity both as a writer and as an inventor (by the way, in case you think him a wimpy intellectual, he also helped start a successful revolt against a world power, risking hanging by the King, and helped start a little club called the United States of America)—when he spoke of his sexual practices helping his creativity, he spoke of why the O-Shot ® changes lives—*sexual energy can fuel boldness and genius.*

Even though philosophers and scientists taught for the past 4,000 years of the benefits of sexual energy used correctly, and even though around ½ of adult women miss these benefits and instead struggle with the life-hampering effects of loss of sexual function, still only 14% of women ever (in their entire life) have a conversation with their physician about sex.

So, some might think it unnecessary to talk about why sex is important but the fact that you're reading this book let's me know that you understand how important sex can be.

An Odd Video Opens My Eyes...

I was lucky enough in medical school to have a class in sexuality, which many medical schools did not have at that time. In the first lecture, on the first day of class, the professor showed a movie of a woman masturbating until she ejaculated.

Then he said, **"I don't want anyone graduating from this medical school thinking that female ejaculation is not real."**

At that time I thought female ejaculation to be an interesting phenomenon, but I didn't realize it would give important clues to female anatomy and physiology that would one day help me understand how to develop the O-Shot ® procedure. So, we'll come back to female ejaculation and how that factors into the O-Shot ®, how it works, and how it's designed.

After some years as an emergency room physician, I opened a private practice in Internal Medicine. I had a researcher's mindset because before medical school I worked 3 years as a research chemist where I developed the and that habit of always looking for the better way and believing there must be a better way. Without that attitude you could not survive as a researcher.

So, though practicing medicine is mostly following standard protocols, I developed the habit of trying to make the protocols better during those years as a research chemist.

When I went into private practice, I decided that one of the primary things needed to keep people healthy would be to help them keep a normal weight. In the United States, most people are overweight; obesity plagues our country with much suffering and death. That's why I began looking for the most advanced thinking on weight loss. So, I found myself in many conferences about weight loss; and when you talk about weight loss, you must talk about hormones.

Hormones control metabolism. Even if you change metabolism by exercising or the way you do your diet (because your diet can increase or slow your metabolism), you're really talking about hormones and how they affect the body and how hormones increase fat storage to make the body obese or increase fat burning to make the body lean.

And of course, *hormones also have much to do with the way people feel and think and how long they live and the health of their brain and their heart—and their sex.*

So, though I was taking care of sick people in the hospital, I decided I really needed to be very good at helping people lose weight. And going down that path as far as I could go led me to a place where I became expert about hormones and pharmaceutical companies hired me to do research. This led to me being flown around the world to meet with other researchers in projects regarding Genotropin and Seizen, two of the brand-name growth hormones.

So, though I started off to help people become very healthy and lose weight, in the process, I talked to over 3000 women in extreme depth about their hormones and their weight—and their sex.

Unexpected Secrets that Lead to Better Sex

To really understand hormones, I found you must talk about sex. Yes, hormones affect weight, hair, digestion, skin, hair, thinking, every body function…but many clues about proper hormone replacement can be found by finding out about sex.

Talking about Hormones Means Talking About Sex

I didn't set out to be extremely knowledgeable about women's sexuality, but if you talk to over 3000 women about their hormones…and also their sex life, then if you prescribe their hormones and you talk to them again and again and again, over a period of years, and you watch how their life changes with what you're doing and what they're doing, *if you do this with over 3,000 women, then you'd have to be stupid not to learn something about women's sexuality. And, I try to not be stupid.*

Over about 10 years' time, working with thousands of women and offering them the best care that I could find, I would talk with them about their sexuality as part of their overall health and they started getting better...

Much Better.

And they got so much better that many of them started outrunning their husbands in the bedroom and then leaving their husbands because they couldn't get the husbands to come see me. The divorce rate in my practice soared, and that bothered me.

So, because many women would cry on their first visit with me because of sexual problems, then (after I treated them) cry in my office because of frustration with the husband who could not keep up with them I wrote a sex book for men. For 3 years, *Anytime...for as Long as You Want* was the best selling sex book on Amazon. Which led to more conversations with men and women who came from all over the world for me to treat them for their sex problems.

But, even though many women improved with the hormone treatments, the urinary incontinence problem did not go away for most. And many women who had normal hormone levels (either because they were young or were already replaced) could not be helped.

Weight Loss Leads to Increased Wrinkles?

The other thing that came out of my work with thousands of women which led to the O-Shot

® was that as the women lost weight, they would complain about their faces. The more weight they lost, as the weight went out of their faces, as the fat left their cheeks, their faces started to droop like a partially deflated balloon. The skin became less tight; wrinkles started to appear that were not there before. Women became happy about their new lean bodies but became depressed about their faces!

"Yes, my body looks younger, more attractive, more shapely, but my face looks older," they would say.

So, in an effort to help that problem, I began searching for the best cosmetic physician injector to teach me the art of facial fillers (like Expressions and Juvederm) so that I could restore the lost volume to a woman's face after she had lost weight. As a result of this cosmetic procedure, she would continue walking and losing weight.

At the time of my search, the top injector in North America (most injections) was Mark Bailey, MD in Toronto, Canada. I visited him several times, spent lots of money and lots of time with him before returning to the United States. Once home, I continued my training, seeking out the best in the country to study and learn from in order to be one of the very best at injecting fillers and Botox to reshape the face so that women would then want to keep losing weight.

That's exactly what happened. Women would lose their 30 or 40 pounds, reward themselves with the cosmetic procedure, and then lose another 30 or 40 pounds.

Because of my educational journey, I developed a then odd combination of skill: (1) expert at hormone replacement, (2) expert at facial injectables, and (3) expert in sexuality.

This combination of skills (sexual medicine, hormones, cosmetic injections) together with a willingness to confess the *5 Critical Confessions of a Sex Doctor* set the stage for the development of the O-Shot ® procedure.

How Blood Can Rejuvenate the Body

Then in 2010, a salesman, John Deeds, walked into my office and told me about lab equipment approved by the FDA for isolating **platelet rich plasma (PRP) from a woman's blood** to put back into her body for rejuvenation of tissue. He explained how it could work similar to an hyaluronic acid filler (like Juvederm, Restylane, and Expressions), and that there had never been a serious side effect—ever.

Next he told me that PRP also increases blood flow with *new blood vessel formation* (not just by dilating the arteries already there).

The result, he said, would be "increased blood flow, new tissue formation (increased volume), and a younger looking face."

So, I thought as a man who had been involved in sex research, "Hmmmm, New blood flow? New Volume? I've got a better place to put PRP than my face."

The idea of NEW blood vessel formation--not simply dilation of blood vessels excited me. Viagra, penile implants, and other current therapies do not create new blood vessels to the penis.

I then searched the medical records and found that John Deeds spoke correctly; I could find no case of serious side effects from PRP. I did, however, find literally thousands of research papers demonstrating the rejuvenation of tissue in bone and skin, and the speeding up of post-surgical healing.

So, I injected faces with PRP for 4 months and invented the Vampire Facelift (R) Procedure and the Vampire Facial Procedure

Out of that experience, I also invented the Vampire Breast Lift ® and the Priapus Shot ® (which helps improve erectile function in men…but that's a subject for another book).

In the process of studying PRP and what it could do in the face and penis, I eventually discovered the O-Shot® procedure. But, before the O-Shot ® could be developed, I had to consider the whole system.

Why I Coined the Phrase "Orgasm System"

There was one other idea that led to the O-Shot ® procedure. In the process of taking care of women who came to me for hormone replacement, I became very angry at how simplified sexuality was considered. There's a **Respiratory System** that involves the lung and the way the air and oxygen exchanges through the lung and into the circulation. There is the **Cardiovascular System** that involves all the blood vessels and the heart and the way it pumps. There's the **Nervous System** that involves the brain and all the peripheral nerves and the spinal column. But female orgasm generation, even female sexuality, seemed to be thought of as this tube called the vagina into which you put a penis that deposits sperm that goes up another tube to the egg.

Because of the hormone practice and the dramatic way my women patients improved their lives, I started to think about the Female Orgasm System. A system is just a collection of different parts and ideas that work together to accomplish a specific purpose. Just as the nervous system involves the brain and the spinal cord and the peripheral nerves and how the synapses of the nerves connect together and how the hormones affect the way the nerves work, the Orgasm System is also a very elaborate and elegant system. The Orgasm System is just as elaborate and just as important as the Nervous System, the Digestive System, and the Cardiovascular System.

What's the advantage of having a system?

Thinking about how the different parts work together, helps understand how to make the whole system work better. For example, if you're trying to make a numb finger regain sensation and you're only thinking about the nerves in the finger (and you're not thinking about the brain or the spinal cord), then you can't really think intelligently about how to make that finger regain sensation. A decrease in sensation of the finger could be from a stroke in the brain, or a lesion in the spinal cord, or a metabolic problem interfering with nerve function, or an anatomical problem with the nerves of the finger.

In the same way, if woman has trouble with sexuality and her sexuality is simplified down to the point of just estrogen and the vagina, then ignoring all the other parts of the orgasm system greatly decreases the chances of finding a solution. For that reason (over simplification and individual-component thinking), many women continue to suffer who could be made well.

The Orgasm System is an elegant integration of multiple anatomical structures, psychological conditions, and hormonal ingredients that work together to create the woman's orgasm— with the resultant pleasure, loving connections, and psychological and creative benefits. To make the system work better, the doctor and the woman need to understand the whole system.

So while I was doing the work with 3,000 plus women and their

16

hormones, I developed a way to think about the Female Orgasm System so that each part can be rejuvenated, enhanced, and tuned to work well with the other parts of the system.

Though I was the first to use the phrase "Female Orgasm System," the phrase came out of the need to think about female sexuality with the same elegance and detail and utility that the other systems of the body are described. *This method of systems analysis can then lead to new methods of healing disease as well as enhancing function to point of bringing disease to a level of super function and intense pleasure and connection.*

So what's in this book?

This book tells how to activate the female orgasm system, the story of how the O-Shot ® procedure came to be, and the stories of women who experienced the O-Shot ® procedure.

In the **first chapter,** we will talk about the **parts of the Orgasm System**: how the brain and the nervous system works to improve orgasm and sexuality, and when I say the orgasm system, I am also thinking about libido and how the orgasm connects people together psychologically and even how it leads to better spirituality and creativity.

So there's the psychology of the orgasm system and the hormones that affect the orgasm.

Also, we will discuss the anatomy of the female genitalia and how that functions to bring a woman pleasure as well as better psychological and physical health.

So in the first chapter of the book we will talk about the Female Orgasm System.

In the **2nd Chapter**, we will talk about **the very 1st O-Shot®
procedure** on the very first woman to experience the shot. How
she and I, alone on the way to a birthday celebration, came upon
the idea.

And then in **Chapter 3** will talk about **how the O-Shot ®
procedure works.** We discuss the science of it, how Dr.
Grofenberg (the original Dr. G), how he thought about the female
anatomy in a much more elegant way than do most modern
physicians in relation to the urethra (and what the G-spot actually
is). We also introduce a new concept: *the O-Spot.*

We talk about ultrasound studies, female ejaculation and the
science behind platelet rich plasma, also how the O-Shot ® is done
and how using the O-Shot ® with other ideas will activate the
female orgasm system.

In the **4ᵗʰ Chapter**, we'll talk about another patient who was **the
second woman to get an O-Shot ® in the world and how it led
her from suffering** (as a single mother in an abusive relationship),
painful intercourse, and poor self esteem **to extremely good sex, a
high self esteem, and a beautiful marriage within a few months.**

In the **5ᵗʰ Chapter**, we talk about **urinary incontinence**, why it
happens, what's available now to make that better, and how the O-
Shot® fits into the possibilities of treatment of urinary
incontinence.

In **Chapter 6**, we go over more **stories about the O-Shot®** and
how sexual dysfunction relates to **childbirth**. We'll talk about
women who experience **ejaculation** for the first time and how that
can happen, why it could be helpful, and why it may not even be
worth thinking about.

And then in the very last chapter, **Chapter 7**, I'll give you ideas
about how to **make a personal plan to tune up your Female**

Orgasm System—step by step-by-step. I'll also outline for each individual problem, what you can do to lead yourself to a place where you can enjoy the pleasure and the social and psychological benefits of a properly functioning orgasm system.

It's maddening to me that people think it's okay to make your digestive system work properly—a good bowel movement in the morning—but nevertheless believe doctors shouldn't think about how to make your Orgasm System work better.

As matter of fact, physicians didn't even describe it as a system until I started writing about the process.

"Let's just call it a vagina, it's just a place to deposit sperm and stick a penis," modern medicine seemed to say.

We can be smarter than that!

So I won't make any apologies about talking about sex and I don't make any apologies about thinking that it's past time that doctors say, "Yes, *there IS a need for thinking about this important bodily function using systems analysis and call it the 'Orgasm System' and we're going to talk about it out loud, and we're going to write about it, and we're going study and work and research about how to make it function better.*"

So that's what we're going to do with this book.

I hope it helps you.

How to Change Your Life

Knowing does not change lives. Doing something different makes a different life. If you suffer with sexual problems or if you'd just like to see you or someone you love enjoy better sex and all the benefits that come from better sex, I hope visit one of the doctors listed at www.OShot.info.

If you can't find the answers you need, I hope you'll write to me. Just know that if the answer's in one of the books I wrote, or if I think there's a doctor that I've trained or worked with that can help you, that's where I'll send you first.

Thank you very much for trusting me enough to pay attention to these ideas about this sacred topic—female sexuality. I'm honored by your interest and I hope that you find the information helpful.

Peace & health,

Charles Runels, MD

Inventor of the O-Shot ® Procedure
http://Runels.com

Doctors should help

Women

Find healthier

And more enjoyable

Sex

By improving the health

Of the

Female Orgasm System.

Chapter 1: Orgasm System Components

The purpose of a system is to do a specific job. The purpose of the circulatory system is to move blood throughout the body. The purpose of the respiratory system is to exchange oxygen, to pull it out of the air and put it into the blood and take carbon dioxide out of the blood and put it back into the air. The circulatory system then delivers that oxygen to all the parts of the body since every part of the body needs oxygen to survive. The nervous system signals movement, senses pleasure and pain, and thinks.

Systems analysis involves thinking about the purpose of the system and then looking at each part of the system as well as how the parts work together in order to make the whole system deliver its purpose in a better way.

Let's start by defining each part of the orgasm system. A rapidly growing body of research describes the system. Each part of the orgasm system could be a whole separate book or a whole lifetime of research. For example, just the anatomy of the vagina or how one part of the brain responds to sexual stimulation can be a whole lifetime of research and has been a lifetime of research for some important researchers.

The following description will be a simplified overview but at least it gives an idea of the different components of the orgasms system. We will talk about one of those components and how it can be rejuvenated by the O-Shot ®. Also, with systems analysis, we'll be able to make a more intelligent plan at the end of this book about how to activate your orgasm system.

Sex Centers in the Physical Brain

The first part of the female orgasm system is the brain. No response, knowledge, pleasure, or benefit takes place without the brain. The brain also controls all the other parts of the orgasm system. Much research for the past 10 years shows which parts of the brain contribute to orgasm.

Research published in May of 2011 showed that to have an orgasm, the woman must become *less aware of the environment*. The woman becomes less aware of the immediate environment as the left hemisphere of the brain becomes deactivated (the *left temporal lobe and the ventral prefrontal cortex*).

Also, now we know that the part of the brain that controls orgasm parallels the part of the brain that controls urination (or micturition): the *dorsolateral pontine area* is active in women who attempted but failed to have an orgasm but the *ventrolateral pontine area* is activated only with ejaculation and orgasm in women [Journal of Sexual Medicine, August of 2013].

Pelvic Organ Stimulating Center

The *pelvic organ stimulating center* (via projections of the sacral parasympathetic motor neurons) controls pelvic organs involved in voiding. The *ventrolateral pontine area* (which is the pelvic force stimulating center) *produces the pelvic contractions during ejaculation in men and physical orgasm in women*. These pathways make only a part of the elaborate system of nerve conduction and brain function that causes orgasm—where one part of the brain deactivates and another part of the brain activates.

Obviously, you don't need to know the names of the parts of the brain to have an orgasm. You'll see later, however, that *it's very important to know that the nerves that control urination cross over with the nerves that control orgasm.*

The Pituitary Gland Conducts the Other Endocrine Glands

Cerebral function controls a part of the brain that also functions as a gland—the pituitary gland. If a woman becomes upset or angry, sleep deprived, or afraid, all these emotions affect the pituitary gland. Then, the pituitary gland controls all of the other glands of the body including the ovaries, testes, and adrenal glands. So, the way a woman thinks will affect her hormones levels!

Psychology: Emotions, Memory, and Feedback Loops

Even though the physical structures like the pituitary gland and left temporal lobe make a major component of the Female Orgasm System, the *woman's psychology must also be considered.* For example, if a woman's left temporal lobe activated as she became acutely aware her surroundings because she's in danger (or worried that the kids are going to walk into the bedroom), then sexual arousal will not elevate to the same level as it would if she grew unaware of the environment (with left temporal lobe deactivating) because she felt safe and comforted.

The effects on sexual function become even more complicated when considering the emotions of love, connection, hate, or resentment.

Psychology of Sex: Fear to Arousal

Fear can be used both to enhance arousal and to dampen arousal in orgasm, depending on what part of the brain senses that fear and how the woman's brain interprets the fear.

If a woman experiences fear and then moves from fear to safety and loss of awareness of environment, the contrasting emotions can heighten sexual arousal. An example would be the sexual arousal that happens after riding a roller coaster or a motorcycle. Emotion and fear form part of what Christian Grey uses to cause the arousal of his lover in *50 Shades of Grey*.

Feedback Loops Set the Stage for Sex

Thinking about psychology in a brain, there's another part of the Female Orgasm System that hasn't been talked about much until fairly recently and that's the idea of a positive or negative feedback loop. In other words, if a woman has a good sexual experience she then looks forward to having sex again and she becomes more easily aroused and achieves a better orgasm and more arousal. On the other hand, if she's frustrated, if she has a sexual experience where she does not have pleasure or she has displeasure or even pain that's uncomfortable and displeasing to her or she becomes aroused and then her lover has premature ejaculation. It's like cranking your car and the engine dies before you leave your driveway. There's a certain amount of frustration.

Then there's a negative feedback loop where the next time she wants to have sex, it becomes more difficult to be aroused. She is anticipating the premature ejaculation or she's anticipating the pain of dyspareunia or the rejection that made her last experience negative. Because of that, she's hesitant and less able to freely experience sexuality and then because of that, she has possibly an even worse experience and so it keeps getting worse and worse instead of better and better.

That positive or negative feedback loop is thought to be very important versus the simplified view that we used to think about or just arousal or plateau orgasm and then after glow. Now we know that it's not individual encounters. Each encounter happens partly based on the things before.

26

Hormone Replacement for Sexual Pleasure

The hormones that affect the Female Orgasm System operate in a more elaborate way than what we thought just a few years ago. Hormones, by definition are chemical messengers that travel through the blood stream to signal other parts of the body. Many of the hormones have receptors on every tissue, meaning the hormone causes a reaction in every tissue type.

Testosterone Needed for Desire and for Orgasm

Testosterone replacement improves both arousal and orgasm in most women. The free testosterone level usually should be replaced to the upper 25% of what's considered normal for a woman.

Methods of replacement include creams, injections, and pellets. I prefer that women start with injections because of absorption is more reliable than creams and the dosage can be adjusted more readily than pellets. After the injection dosage is perfected, then the woman may be swapped to one of the other methods if she prefers after the proper dosage for response and blood levels have been determined by injection. Not just the total but also the free testosterone, which is unbound of protein and the biologically active part of testosterone, should be checked. If a woman has not had a free testosterone level done, there's no way to intelligently tune up her orgasm system.

Thyroid Does Much More Than Keep You Thin

Thyroid is extremely important and this idea of what's normal is becoming more debated as normal levels for lab tests are determined by doing a bell curve. To determine normal levels, researchers find normal people, test them, and then find the average just like back when back in school. The F's and the A+'s are loped off and somewhere in between that's what's called "normal."

If you're trying to give people optimal function, why would you call something normal that's a C or a D and not move them up into the higher level of what's considered to be normal if that higher level indeed causes a higher level of function?

But, not every hormone should be adjusted to the high end of normal. Though high-normal levels of testosterone and thyroid may lead to a thinner, healthier body and high sex drive, estrogen, can be carcinogenic and cause weight gain and bloating; so most women seem healthier if estrogen stays on the lower end of normal. Many people think that replacing estrogen will help sex drive, but estrogen does little for sex drive. Primarily, estrogen serves to help with memory, emotional attachment, female body characteristics, and vaginal mucosal health.

Thyroid receptors can be found on every tissue type: for example the skin, the brain, the gut, and the heart. That's why if thyroid is too high, the heart will go too fast, people lose body fat and they feel nervous; but, if thyroid levels fall too low, the woman feels sleepy and gains body fat while the heart beats too slowly.

There are literally receptors to react to the thyroid level and receive that message on every part of the body. You get constipated if thyroid's too low. The bowel has receptors.

The same thing applies with testosterone—receptors on every tissue type. Understanding how to replace these hormones and doing it properly involves a very sophisticated look at how the body functions. Proper hormone replacement requires keeping track of what happens with a woman's body (including the sexual response) as well as keeping track of blood levels.

Growth hormone has been shown to have a profound effect on body weight, feelings of well being, of outgoingness, and of mental focus. With men, growth hormone affects firmness of erection. With women, profoundly affects sense of well-being to the point where if it's low, people are more likely to feel depressed and tired and achy which of course would interfere with the emotions of arousal and libido and orgasm. So, growth hormone levels should definitely be measured, usually by checking IGF-1 (insulin-like growth factor 1).

Unfortunately, growth hormone became a politically charged hormone. I think beyond its level of risk, it's not even listed as a carcinogenic on the FDA-approved drug profile and yet it has a reputation of being dangerous. People, who have levels of growth hormone that are too high, acromegalics, have 25% less cancer than the general population. Studies of children with low pituitary function with decreased growth hormone secondary to surgery for pituitary cancer, these children see less recurrence of their brain cancer when their growth hormone is replaced.

So, growth hormone probably protects against cancer, yet it has this bad rap and bad laws that make doctors afraid to prescribe it even though it's extremely beneficial. At least in the US it's become a really politically charged hormone, which makes it difficult to even do good medicine anymore. Hopefully that will change soon.

Prolactin

Prolactin causes breast milk production. If it's too high, a woman will produce breast milk even if she's not pregnant. If prolactin levels are too high, it can cause feelings of lack of arousal, decreased libido, and difficulty with orgasm so it should be checked. It's one of the hormones that you want to keep on the low side. If it's too high, then there's a pill that can be taken (Dostinex) to lower the levels.

Estrogen

Estrogen really bothers me because we know it's potentially carcinogenic. Estrogen also leads to weight gain, but it helps people look like women so it's a useful thing.

Estrogen also helps keep the vaginal mucosa healthy, helps with thinking and memory but estrogen does not really help with libido. It can help with feelings of attachment and the feelings of emotions of love and tenderness but as far as making the sex more passionate and improving the sex drive and orgasm, it just does not contribute.

It's better kept on the lower end of normal, not abnormally low, but the lower end of normal. Many of my patients, if they're post-menopausal, they get all the estrogen they need simply from the conversion of the testosterone, part of testosterone gets converted to estrogen by the liver.

Progesterone

Research shows that progesterone helps protect the breasts and the uterus from cancer by down regulating estrogen receptors. Progesterone affects the libido more than estrogen but less than testosterone.

The idea that all hormones are dangerous is just wrong. You need hormone to stay alive! Hormone can even help protect from cancer as well as support the heart and the brain.

So, we've looked at some of the major hormones, but the pituitary gland make more than 230 hormones that we know about so far! So the idea of just giving the woman estrogen or a little testosterone and not following levels is really so primitive that it saddens me that women still receive such treatment. Hormones should be thought of in a much more sophisticated level and with the idea that even if you do all these blood levels it's still very primary compared to the way body actually works.

Thankfully, hormone chain reactions happen—so if you give a woman testosterone, it decreases her thyroid binding globulin and effectively raises her functioning thyroid. If you give her growth hormone, it helps her testosterone work better, and on and on. You can't change one hormone without changing other hormones. I'm sure there are chain reactions we don't yet understand when you consider just the 200 plus hormones made by the pituitary gland and the 6 hormones made by the thyroid.

Oxytocin for Love

The pituitary gland normally releases oxytocin when the woman delivers a baby. This hormone causes uterine contraction therefore helping stop bleeding from the uterus after the child is delivered. Oxytocin also causes feelings of tenderness and love toward the child.

Massage and orgasm also increase oxytocin levels. Some people make less oxytocin just like some make less of the other hormones. Just like some people are taller than others or have different colored eyes or different size ring fingers, they make different amounts of oxytocin. Research shows that lower levels of oxytocin can be found in women who experience fewer emotions of love and tenderness with orgasm.

Oxytocin and growth hormone (unlike thyroid, estrogen, and testosterone) are small proteins—short chains of amino acids. Think of each amino acid like a links in a chain where the chain makes the protein and the order of that chain makes the message (defines the hormone).

If you arrange certain amino acids in one way, you have insulin. You arrange them in another way, you have oxytocin or growth hormone.

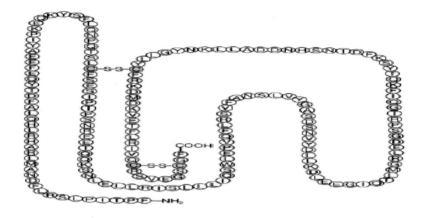

Because the stomach contains acid, these protein hormones cannot be taken by mouth and be effective because the acid digests or breaks the chains into individual amino acids (digestion) so the individual amino acids can be absorbed. Digestion of protein would be like giving you a word and then having the word broken into individual letters by the stomach because the stomach cannot absorb the whole word.

The hormone makes the word that delivers the message. For example, oxytocin travels from the pituitary gland to deliver the message to the brain to cause feelings of tenderness and to deliver the message to the uterus to cause muscle contraction (both good things if you're having sex). But if you take oxytocin by mouth, then nothing happens because the stomach digests the protein oxytocin into the individual amino acids. Then the body just sees the same amino acids as if you simply ate a hamburger because the word (hormone) broke apart into individual letters (amino acids).

Hormone Traps

One quick warning: Some will try to fool you and sell the protein hormones like growth hormone and oxytocin as a pill. You can be sure that you cannot get growth hormone or prolactin or oxytocin as a tablet because you cannot get insulin that way (since insulin is also a small protein and you can be sure that the best technology will be used to take care of diabetics). When you see diabetics able to take insulin as a pill, you will then know that you can get growth hormone as a pill.

As of now, you can get the protein hormones like growth hormone, insulin, and oxytocin as an injection or a nasal spray since both of these routes go around the acid in the stomach.

Yes, there's insulin that's a nasal spray. Most people prefer the injections for these hormones though because it's such a tiny needle that only needs to go under the skin (not into the muscle) and that's what I recommend with growth hormone and oxytocin if your levels test low.

Another big trap: women on birth control pills will drop their testosterone levels as a side effect of the birth control pills. This drop in testosterone can then lead to weight gain, migraines, and decreased sexual function. In a typical scenario, a young woman delivers a child and then starts taking birth control pills. She thinks the decreased sex drive weight gain that follows comes from having had a baby but it's often from the effects of the birth control pills. Sometimes the pills can be adjusted out to correct the problem; sometimes she needs to take a little testosterone while she's on the pill and just come off of the testosterone when she comes off of the birth control pill.

In summary, hormones are a huge part of the orgasm system and proper hormone balance requires careful attention to both

blood levels and the woman's symptoms. A woman will struggle to have a sex drive or an orgasm without proper hormone balance.

Blood Flow Increases Arousal and Orgasm

The Female Orgasm System also depends upon circulation. Blood flows to the brain, the vagina, the breasts, and to other parts of the body from the toes to the scalp—all of which have erotic capabilities. Circulation can be changed with respiration, hormones, and cardiac function. Techniques can be used with breath control that both enhance or inhibit the orgasm response.

The blood flow to the vagina supports arousal and orgasm.

Skene's Glands

Now we know that women who ejaculate (versus urinate) with sex actually excrete fluid from small glands near the opening of the urethra called the **Skene's glands** or **periurethral glands**. These glands make a fluid that we now know contains some of the same chemical components as prostate (prostate specific antigen). So, these glands in a woman excrete fluid like that from the prostate of a man. These glands can be found near the opening of the urethra, not back where the urethra joins the bladder.

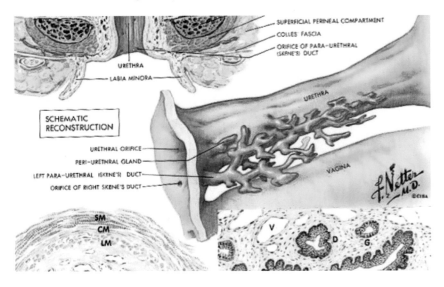

Urethra

Dr. Gräfenberg (for whom the G-Spot is named) thought the urethra the most erotic part of a woman's body. Stimulating the G-spot means simply pushing against the roof of the vagina where the urethra lies just on the other side of the vaginal wall. If a woman lies supine, it would be the top or the front of the vagina. Since that's where the urethra is, putting pressure there causes sexual stimulation. The area specifically near where the urethra joins the bladder was thought by Dr. Gräfenberg to be the most erotic part of the urethra.

Nerve Tissue to Support Sex

Another part of the Female Orgasm System anatomy includes the peripheral nerves (the nerves outside the brain in the body). The peripheral nerves of the orgasm system include not just the nerves that detect sensation and control musculature of the vaginal wall but also the nerves of every other part of the body: the back, the neck, the feet, the mouth, the hands, the breast, every part of the body. All the nerves of the body connect back to the brain where ideas of sexual arousal and orgasm can be found.

Dr. Gräfenberg, even though he was THE Dr. "G" and described the G-Spot, **considered every part of a woman's body to be erotic**. Every part of the body can be erotic and contribute to the orgasm system.

So, *any therapy or idea that enhances sensation of any part of the body could contribute to enhancing the orgasm system!*

The Hidden Secret Part of the Clitoris

Most people think of the clitoris as the part that you can see. But, the clitoris is mostly inside the body. The visible part correlates to the glans (or head) of the penis. But, most of the clitoris, the part that correlates to the shaft of the penis, lies hidden inside the woman's   body.

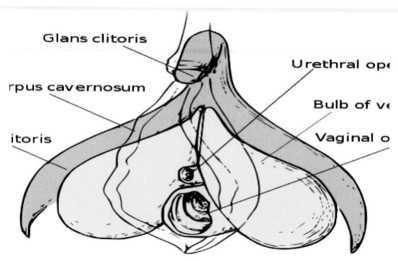

What if *only* the glans of a man's penis was stimulated and not the shaft? What if during sexual intercourse, only the glans was allowed within the vagina and not the shaft? He would experience pleasure but he would probably experience more pleasure if the shaft were stimulated too.

The same idea applies to the woman! Now we know that the inner part of the clitoris comes close to the roof of the vagina with stimulation. A woman routinely has a clitoris 5 or 6 inches long; you're only seeing the tip of it on the outside.

Later, I'll explain a way to rejuvenate and activate the inside part of the clitoris.

Vagina: The Least Sensitive Part

There's also of course the vagina itself, the mucosa surface of the vagina, and the musculature of the vagina. The vaginal wall senses touch and pressure much less than does the urethra, the clitoris, or the anus. To help understand, the clitoris is analogous to the penis and the labia would have been the scrotum; both of these structures bring pleasure to a man when stimulated, but which is the most sensitive? And, so it is with the female.

Other Parts of the Female Orgasm System

The rectum also relates to the vaginal sensation. The cervix, the ovaries, and the uterus should also be considered. All of those parts of the anatomy are important to the Female Orgasm System.

In the next chapter, we'll talk about the very first O-Shot ®; then, in Chapter 3, we'll show how I designed the O-Shot ® procedure based on the parts of the Female Orgasm System that we just described.

Chapter 2: The Very First O-Shot ® Ever—Anywhere

On the evening of April first, 2011, I drove through Fairhope, Alabama to pick up my girlfriend from her house to take her to dinner for her birthday. As we were preparing to leave her house to go to dinner, she said, "I want PRP injected into my vagina!"

Why a Woman Asked for Her Blood to Be Injected Into Her Vagina

As you know from the introduction to this book, PRP (or platelet rich plasma) comes from a person's own blood (autologous) and can be used to stimulate multipotent stem cells to rejuvenate new tissue.

But, why would a woman decide she wants a shot in the vagina using her own blood!?

For the past year, Laura had watched me inject people and rejuvenate the face and the breasts. She actually had the procedure done more than once and saw her face improve in color, texture, and shape with a procedure I invented, the Vampire Facelift ®.

Also, she had regained sensation in her breasts (which she had lost due to breast implants and breastfeeding 3 children) with a procedure I designed called the Vampire Breast Lift ®.

She had delivered 3 children and wanted to see if PRP would make her vagina feel tighter. Also, she was able to have an orgasm but still had some difficulty with multiple orgasms and wanted to see if the PRP would help tighten her vagina and improve her orgasms.

I thought since there are no known serious side effects from the use of PRP anywhere in the body (and there are thousands of research papers), "We'll try it and see what happens."

I took her to the office.

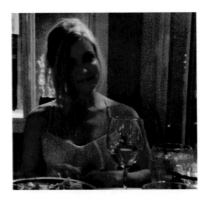

To isolate platelet rich plasma (PRP), I drew blood from her arm (just like if she were giving blood at the laboratory for a test).

As part of the strategy of where to put the injection, I ideas that I explain in a book I wrote about how to teach women to understands her body better and become able to ejaculate. I had already taught Laura to ejaculate, but placed part of the PRP in the areas most responsible for this response (more about that in the next chapter).

I drew Laura's blood and centrifuged it. Then, I added the calcium chloride, which is like salt water (sodium chloride), only calcium instead of sodium. The calcium chloride signals the platelets that there's been a tissue injury.

Usually, calcium concentrations in tissue exceed those in the blood. When tissue sustains an injury, then calcium's released from the injured tissue. When calcium, which is normally in the lower concentration in the blood stream, becomes higher in concentration in the blood, then the platelets "think," "Oh, there's been an injury! Let's signal for repair to start."

Then the thrombin cascade activates causing a clot that stops the bleeding. The platelets also release at least 7 powerful growth factors that we know about so far (there could be more). These growth factors stimulate multipotent stem cells to rejuvenate the tissue.

For the past 15 years, dentists, surgeons, and veterinarians have used this process to rejuvenate tissue and promote healing post operation and after trauma. These specialists use PRP for orthopedic surgery of the knees, in dental surgery to help healing, and rejuvenate the knees of elite thoroughbred racehorses.

If you want to know what works, look at what the NFL does to keep their athletes going. If someone's making 10 million dollars a year and they miss a day of work that's sort of expensive. One of the things they do is use platelet rich plasma to rejuvenate the tissue of the joints. Why shouldn't a woman enjoy the same rejuvenating benefits that help an elite athlete run down the football field to help her develop a healthier body—including improvement of the vaginal tissue needed for sex and urination?

Also, since physicians have been searching for over 15 years for something that can be injected around the urethra to cure urinary incontinence, I knew from that research that putting a needle in the vaginal area is safe (previous attempts to discover a method gave side effects not from the needle but from the material injected). A much larger needle than I intended to use in that area can be used to drain the bladder with no ill effects from the needle.

Knowing that PRP also causes no side effects and that needles in that area cause no serious injury, I thought, "Okay, it could work!

I'll possibly give her the same rejuvenation benefits enjoyed by the NFL and racehorses (new healthier tissue) if I give her PRP in the vagina."

I gave her the shot and in the process of doing that, I went ahead and injected some of that plasma where I knew Laura collected fluid when she ejaculated.

I did not even need a speculum; all the important structures I wanted to rejuvenate can be easily seen near the opening of the vagina with nothing more than a strong lamp.

I also thought, "While I'm at it (knowing the anatomy of the vagina and knowing that most of the clitoris is within the body and knowing how plasma behaves like water) I'll inject the part of the clitoris that's visible and hopefully rejuvenate the whole structure."

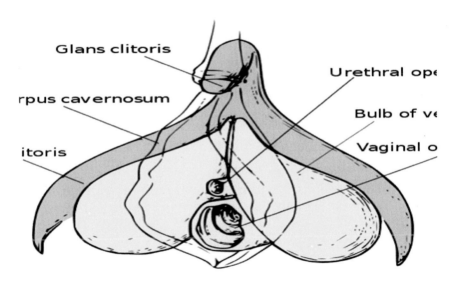

When I injected her clitoris, rather than the clitoris swelling out, as expected, the fluid disappeared within Laura's body, travelling into each side of the inner clitoris. I couldn't see it but I could see that a much greater volume than what was exposed of the clitoris was actually injected into it—yet the clitoris did not expand, it just absorbed. The PRP had to go somewhere and observation was that it was going into the depths of her clitoris to rejuvenate that tissue.

After the procedure, Laura put her dress back on and we went to dinner. I expected maybe 2-3 weeks later she might see some benefit.

Her body would give me a huge surprise.

The Big O Surprise

The next day, Laura texted, "I can't stop masturbating! I'm still in bed! That shot made things go crazy down there!!!! ;) "

I looked at my watch; it was 12:30 PM.

Although her reaction interested me, I grew puzzled over the fact that her response happened before the stem cells could actually grow new tissue.

Why?

Before I tell you my hypothesis about what happened, think back to Dr. Gräfenberg. He thought that every part of a woman's body is potentially erotic and I agree with that. But, he thought of the whole female body, the most erotic part is the urethra.

Having worked in the emergency room in the past, I remember seeing x-ray photographs where women lost little things up in the urethra because they put them in the urethra for sexual stimulation

Dr. Gräfenberg thought encouraged stimulating the urethra through the roof of the vagina by manual pressure and particularly in the part where the urethra joins the bladder. From that idea came the "The G-spot" (named after Dr. Gräfenberg).

Where I gave the shot was more proximal than the area usually considered the G-Spot: between the vaginal wall and the urethra at the spot where the Skene's glands collect fluid.

That *space* **between the two structures (urethra and vagina), near the opening of the vagina, needed a name...so I called it the "O-Spot."**

That's where I injected the PRP, in the O-Spot.

When a woman ejaculates, the fluid from the Skene's glands is what accounts for the fluid that comes from her body. We now know from ultrasound studies and from biochemical analyses that the "female prostate," the Skene's glands (just like the prostate gland of men) contributes to the fluid of the ejaculate by excreting fluid into the urethra. The fluid from the Skene's glands even tests positive for prostate specific antigen (PSA), normally considered being associated only with men!

Just as different men might have different sized prostate glands, so might a woman have more or less Skene's glands? I postulated that when I injected the vagina, it might help this tissue become healthier and enhance pleasure and perhaps even enhance ejaculation. So, I placed the injection where I knew to be the location of Laura's Skene's glands.

Why would a woman enjoy more pleasure if she develops more or healthier glandular tissue?

Roller Coasters & Vaginas

Consider riding a roller coaster: you're going to experience more of a thrill if there's a longer fall from a taller hill. In the same way, arousal and orgasm will be heightened if the fluid that's released is increased in volume. Relief of sexual tension (orgasm) feels enhanced if the sexual tension is enhanced with more fluid.

It turns out that Laura's hyper-sexuality (which was almost a nuisance to her because of the extreme intensity) went away by the end of the first week. Even though Laura was very sexual before the shot, it became extremely urgent for her to have sex and orgasms grew more intense and more powerful right from the start. Then it faded some just like we've seen when we inject platelet rich plasma into other tissue.

The more long lasting effects started to appear around the third week as those multipotent stem cells grew new tissue. We know from biopsy studies of other parts of the body that new tissue includes fibroblast and glandular tissue and bone and whatever happens to be there.

In the skin, where there are fat cells, the fat cells enlarge and multiply. The best way to think about PRP: it's like that yellow goo that was around the scab when you scraped your knee when you fell as a child. You had to grow new skin to replace what had been peeled away when you fell. And it's that yellow goo around the scab where the growth factors are embedded; that's what I was making when I injected the plasma into Laura's vagina.

Three weeks later, she indeed became even more easily aroused and although the hyper-sexuality of needing sex continuously was relieved, when we did have sex, it felt tighter us both and her ejaculations became *much more intense*, her orgasms became more easily achieved, and vaginally-produced orgasms (with penis-in-vagina) became more easily found.

You might think, "Well, this is sort of like trick circus sex, where a shot somehow makes a woman able to do something that she wasn't able to do."

Some people think of female ejaculation as just a little extra trick. It's much more than that. It's about having a healthy body, every part of the body, including the genitals at full function.

A mountain of research supports the idea that there's a different type of connection with different types of orgasm. If sex makes a connection between people that establishes relationships like families and marriage and love, then that supports people. If you believe that love and relationships and connections are important and that sex somehow contributes to those connections, then I think it might make sense that it's worth while to do something with a woman's own natural growth factors to encourage healing and enhancement of that natural health and that way of connecting—through sexuality.

When I began offering this procedure to my patients, I called it the "O-Shot®" or "Orgasm Shot®" and trademarked the name to keep the rare quack from misleading people with the name. A few months later, I started teaching the procedure to other physicians.

Only certified physicians can legally use the name. Others may make PRP and inject it, but there's a wide variation in how the PRP can be made; at last count, there's 19 lab kits approved by the FDA for preparation of PRP for injection back into the body--all of them working a little differently. Also, there could be a very wide variation in how the injection can be done!

To complicate things, though the FDA controls the kits that are offered to physicians for preparation of PRP, the FDA does not control how blood products are used. Since, only the woman's blood (no drug) is used in the procedure, it seemed helpful to me to control those who can offer the procedure so that a standard of excellence could be established and enforced.

So, Laura was the first to receive the O-Shot ® procedure ever in the world and I'm forever grateful (and many women will also be grateful) to Laura for her courage to want to be the first.

Remember, only 14% of women in their entire life, by a recent study published in obstetrics and gynecology, ever have a conversation with their physician about sex even though 40-60% of them have problems that seriously bother them. Research shows that physicians try to avoid the subject because they don't (not yet) have general knowledge of the O-Shot ® and the ways to help with sexual problems.

Everyone seems to avoid even discussing sex problems with women. Surprisingly even some of the sex therapists (surprisingly even women sex therapists) seem to criticize women who want to experience better sexual health that includes the help of a physician.

So, it took a combination of Laura's courage and trust in me as well as my understanding of female sexual function and anatomy to conceive of the procedure.

Another Woman (*Not* Another Doctor)

I treated around 20 other women over the next 2 months before finally offering to teach the procedure to other physicians. Some have tried to claim helping think of the procedure, but I want to make sure everyone knows—this life changing procedure came about NOT because of help from another physician. No other physician helped me think of this idea though many will research it in the future. Nope...that's not fair to Laura! The only other person who helped me think of this procedure was a very courageous woman, *Laura Ezekiel*, by volunteering to be the first patient.

A Plea for YOUR Help to Relieve 50 Million Women of Their Pain

I hope that you will open the idea that whatever is available to help an NFL athlete run faster to carry a football (PRP) should be considered at least (and offered when appropriate) to women who might want to have more sexual pleasure and better vaginal health. This is not mutilation, this is not even surgery, there is no scalpel, there is no foreign body; this is a woman's own natural healing factors, from her own body. With the O-Shot® procedure, the physician uses the same factors that woman's body used to heal a scraped knee when she was young girl.

Why shouldn't a 50-year old woman who's trying to maintain the relationship with her husband and avoid peeing on her leg when she goes for a walk or when she coughs at work—why shouldn't she have that same technology available to her that's available to an Olympic athlete or a thoroughbred horse?

I'm begging you to not attack the women who display the courage to try this new therapy and I'm begging you to ask your gynecologists to look carefully at the science behind the procedure.

Because this is not a drug, this procedure is not something where there's millions of dollars available for research. There's no attractive woman sales person that's going to walk into gynecologist's office and say, "Dr. Jones, you should prescribe this." And, since this procedure involves only the woman's own blood, all of the research efforts thus far were financed by the physicians listed at www.OShot.info.

I promise you that if a drug that could do what the O-Shot ® procedure does, this would be all over your TV and you'd be seeing commercials about it—but because there's no drug company with millions of dollars to be made, and because insurance doesn't yet pay for it, most doctors don't know about it—*NOT YET!*

The first heart catheterization was done in the 1940's and the doctor was kicked out of the hospital and got so depressed, he wound up in an insane asylum even though he had the courage to do the first heart cath on himself. But, the heart catheterization wasn't commonly done until the 1970's—30 years later.

Do not let that happen with the O-Shot ® procedure.

On average, it takes 10 years to prove a new therapy in medicine. Then, once it's proven, once you have one research study, and people attack it then there's more research. New things in medicine evolve with a very gradual acceptance as more research is done.

Then surprisingly, many physicians still won't offer a new therapy unless insurance pays for it because they don't have enough time (they're working so hard already) to do things for free.

So, usually 10 years passes before the herd of sheep-physicians finally say, "Okay, we can start now, since this is proven."

Then another 10 years passes before the whole herd starts doing the new procedure. So usually it takes10 years to prove a new therapy and another 10 years before it's commonly done – 20 years total from conception to common use.

Please help shorten this time frame with the O-Shot ® procedure. Please consider the 50 million women in the US alone who need this for sexual function and 20 million women in the US who need it for urinary incontinence.

Question: Do you know the number one reason for a women going to a nursing home?

Answer: It's urinating on the floor because...the family will keep grandmother at home even with dementia, even with frailty; but when grandmother can't hold her urine, then she becomes a hygiene problem and too much work.

So, when grandmother can't get to the bathroom without urinating on the floor, that is the most common reason for finally giving up and putting her in the nursing home. Because the O-Shot ® will usually stop urinary incontinence without the side effects of anti-cholinergic medicines and the risks of surgery, this represents a breakthrough in women's health. For the sake of all the grandmothers, I'm pleading: think about it, look at it, convince yourself; then show your friends and your doctor the website and blog and text about it: www.OShot.info .

In Chapter 4, I'll tell you the story of O-Shot ® number 2 (about a woman who was cured of severe pain). But first, in the next chapter, let's look more closely at how the O-Shot ® procedure works.

Chapter 3: How the O-Shot ® Works

The science behind the O-Shot ® started with Dr. Gräfenberg. We spoke earlier about how he thought that the urethra was the most erotic part of a woman's body. Even though every part of a woman's body can be stimulated in such a way to be sexually arousing, the intensity of arousal and the way the urethra contributes to orgasm is particularly powerful.

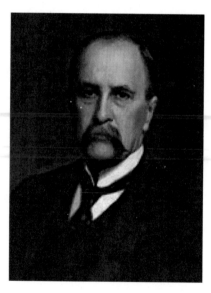

Dr. Ernst Gräfenberg for whom the G-Spot Is named (arrested in Nazi Germany because he was a Jew, fled to the US)

Now we know what Dr. Gräfenberg didn't know and that is how the innervation of the brain with micturition or urination cross-innervates with that orgasm all through the urethra.

We also now know through ultrasound studies that the space between the urethra and the vagina near the opening of the vagina only measures about a 1/4 of an inch thick in an 18-year-old woman. Also, from ultrasound, we know that the thicker that space is (the O-Spot), the more easily a woman can have a vaginal orgasm.

In women who ejaculate, ultrasound studies show that the fluid is coming from glandular tissue that surrounds the urethra in the same way that the prostate gland surrounds the urethra of a male. That tissue, those glands are called the periurethral glands or Skene's glands. They're very close to the opening of the urethra where the water actually comes out. By ultrasounds studies that fluid is secreted from the glands into the urethra then out of the woman's body when she ejaculates.

The Magic Elixir Waiting in the Blood

The other science that allowed the development of the O-Shot ® is that of platelet rich plasma (PRP). People have been doing research for 20 years looking at ways to extract growth factors from the blood stream—the same growth factors that stimulate wound healing when someone sustains and injury—and use them to promote healing after surgery or to help healing from disease. For instance, studies demonstrate taking this platelet rich plasma and putting it into the knee will help rejuvenate cartilage.

Also, thousands of studies looking at wound care. For example, if someone suffers with skin that's been pulled away by trauma to the point to where not enough skin remains to cover the bone of the foot and ankle, there are studies demonstrating that platelet rich plasma helps regrow skin over the bone.

Also, when someone undergoes heart bypass surgery, the breastbone (sternum) heals slowly and can become more easily infected because of decreased blood supply. Research shows that

platelet rich plasma (the same material used in the O-Shot®
procedure) propagates healing of the sternum and helps protect
against infection.

Biopsy studies (where doctors injected PRP into the skin and then
a few weeks later sampled pieces of that skin to look at under the
microscope) show new collagen, new blood vessel formation, and
enlargement of multiplication of fat cells with no abnormal cell
formation. Using these ideas, I first started using platelet rich
plasma (PRP) to rejuvenate the tissue of the face in a procedure
that I invented called the Vampire Facelift ®: "Vampire" to
indicate the use of blood and "Facelift" to indicate restoring
volume to the face in the proper areas—lifting tissue away from
the bone to restore the youthful shape and glow of a young person.

The knowledge gained in the development of the Vampire
Facelift® procedure (how the PRP can be prepared and how it
behaves and works when injected into the body) prepared me for
the idea of how to design the O-Shot® procedure.

Preparing the Magic Elixir

The process of preparing PRP takes only a few minutes right in the
room with the patient.

First, the doctor or nurse places blood in a centrifuge. The
centrifuge spins at about 3,000 RPM's. At this speed, the heaviest
parts of the blood (the red blood cells) go to the bottom and the
lightest parts of the blood (the platelets) are left at the top.

The doctor then activates the plasma using a small amount of
calcium and the platelet rich plasma (PRP) starts to turn into a
gel—platelet rich fibrin matrix (PRFM).

PRFM will not pass through a needle because it is very thick. So,
within minutes of activating the PRP with calcium, it must be

injected—then the PRP turns into PRFM within the woman's body and that holds the growth factors in place to rejuvenate that area of tissue.

Is It Safe?

The medical research contains no reports of serious side effects from PRP prepared with an FDA approved kit EVER! (The FDA has approved about 20 different lab kits for this purpose). I know of no other medical procedure where this is the case. When you think about it thought, it makes sense that PRP would be safe. Platelet rich plasma is derived from the woman's own bloodstream. There's no foreign body to react to. And PRP is what the body would make to heal from other procedures!

I didn't invent the process of preparing PRP; I just designed ways to use PRP to rejuvenate the face (Vampire Facelift®) and vaginal tissue (O-Shot® procedure).

I'm Not the First Person to Put a Needle in the Vagina

The other part of the science that prepared the way for the O-Shot®: for the past 20 years, people have been injecting material around the urethra to try to treat urinary incontinence.

One material tried and still used is called calcium hydroxyapatite crystals. They're used in the face to help restore volume in the face; the brand name for the material used in the face is Radiesse.

Even though Radiesse works beautifully in the face for restoring volume, if a doctor puts Radiesse in lip he's in danger of malpractice because it's very likely that the patient will develop a hard, lumpy granuloma. The crystals stimulate volume by being resorbed and work safely in deep tissue like the cheek; but as the crystals resorb—if placed in a thin mucosal surface like the lip or vagina—the incidence of granuloma goes up dramatically. When this material's placed around the urethra, a granuloma can cause a blockage severe enough to block the woman's urethra completely. So, the woman can't urinate at all without emergency surgery!

One in 40 people (in one study) who have calcium hydroxyapatite crystals placed around the urethra (even though it's an FDA approved in a material similar to Radiesse called Coaptite) will have a granuloma that's so significant and severe that it must be surgically removed.

The useful knowledge that came out of the research with Coaptite is that even though the material used proved less than desirable, the idea of using a needle there proved very safe (even though the needle used to place Coaptite is much larger than the needle used for the O-Shot ® procedure. The size needle that we use for the O-Shot ® could be put into the carotid artery without causing problems and larger needles are used to drain the bladder of little children who suffer with a blockage of the urethra.

Even putting material in the vaginal wall to improve sexual function has been tried, using a material like Juvederm or hyaluronic acid (HA) filler (or "collagen").

Putting these materials there for improved sexual function (but not for treatment of dysfunction) was popularized under a different name. The idea promoted was to create a bump at the G-spot so that the penis rubs against it more. With this method, there's NO rejuvenation involved, only increased friction by causing more volume right where the G-spot is.

I studied the work of physicians who tried injecting HA fillers and collagen, and crystals as part of research for developing the O-

Shot® procedure. Injecting HA fillers in this way is thought to be so dangerous that that shot has been condemned by the American College of Gynecology in the United States of America. There are just too many women who suffered problems with granulomas that had to be removed surgically as a side effect of the procedure.

The idea of injecting around the urethra was not condemned; the previous materials (prior to the O-Shot ®) used were just not safe enough. Also, the location and method differed in slight but important ways from the O-Shot® procedure.

That's the science of the O-Shot ® procedure. Let's get to the actual mechanics of how the procedure is done and you'll see how the science is put into action.

What Happens When You Get the O-Shot® Procedure

First, the doctor will want to know details about the woman's health and sexual history.

Then, the provider helps the patient apply a numbing cream. There's no reason to have pain even with phlebotomy, so numbing cream is applied to the woman's arm (where the needle will be used to draw blood) and the numbing cream is applied to the vaginal mucosa near the opening as well as to the clitoris. The numbing cream is a special mixture of 3 strong numbing agents mixed in a cream that promotes rapid and complete absorption into the mucosa of the vagina.

The provider draws blood (a couple of tablespoons) from the woman's arm and places the blood into a container in a centrifuge.

The centrifuge exaggerates gravity. When gravity increases, then the heavier parts of the blood go towards the bottom and the lighter components stay near the top of the container.

The lightest part of the blood is the platelets. If you let the centrifuge go with the right of time and the right speed, you can extract the platelets.

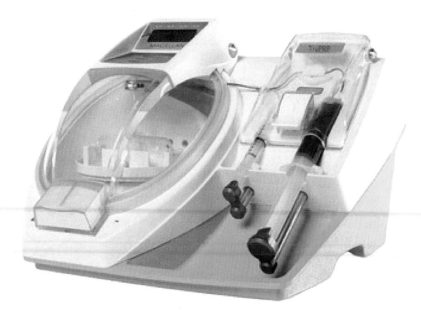

The kits need to be FDA-approved because if you're going to process blood to put it back into the body, that's a much more tricky thing than just processing it to do a lab test and analyze a blood level. I could analyze your blood and find out wonderful things about it but make it unacceptable, even not sterile enough, to be put back into your body.

So, the FDA does and should approve kits for processing blood to put back into the body either for a transfusion or, in this case, for isolation and use of platelet derived growth factors. Some physicians process blood without using one of these FDA approved kits and that should not be done. Not using an FDA approved kit risks infection and can cause too much variability in the platelet concentration.

When you see a physician who's doing the O-Shot ® for you, she should be using an FDA-approved kit.

Activation of Blood/Platelets to Release Rejuvenation Factors

Normally, blood contains more sodium than calcium. With tissue damage, for example a crush injury or a laceration here's what happens:

a) The injured tissue releases calcium.

b) Calcium signals to the platelets that there's been an injury.

c) Platelets respond by activating the thrombin cascade.

d) The thrombin cascade causes a blood clot (partly from the platelet rich fibrin matrix--PRFM) and stops the bleeding. PRFM is the yellow goo you saw around your scab on your knee when you fell as a child.

e) Platelets release growth factors into the matrix, which holds the growth factors in place.

f) Growth factors stimulate and recruit multipotent stem cells to grow new, healthier tissue.

The Elixir Placed Where Needed

By now (after the blood has centrifuge), the woman can feel very little in the vaginal area due to the effects of the numbing cream.

Then, the provider uses a very thin needle (same size used in the face and mouth with cosmetic procedures) to inject in a VERY SPECIFIC WAY a teaspoon of the PRP (which is now turning into PRFM) into the roof of the vagina.

About 1/5 of a teaspoon also goes into the clitoris.

The woman will be comfortable with the injection to the vagina and most will feel no pain with the injection to the clitoris. Some people will feel the injection of the clitoris with slight pain (but the pain will be greatly diminished by the numbing cream).

When it's injected, that material travels through the clitoris, it's like injecting a sponge. If you took a needle and injected water into a sponge, it wouldn't just stay in one spot—the water would be absorbed through the sponge. In the same way, when you inject the clitoris, you don't see the clitoris expand, it stays about the same size and the material just disappears as it's absorbed into that deeper part of the clitoris where most of it lies unseen on each side of the vagina within the woman's body. If the clitoris responds like the rest of the body does, the knee, the mouth, the sternum, the skin then it's going to be rejuvenated with better blood flow, better sensation and overall healthier tissue. The same thing would happen to the roof of the vagina.

So, when we put PRP between the vaginal wall and the urethra, think what's going to happen: new fibroblast activity and rejuvenation of the glands that produce the fluid that lubricates the vaginal wall. Also, libido should go up in the same way that a man might have increased libido if the seminiferous tubules or the prostate gland becomes boggy with collection of fluid to the point of sort of increasing the urge to ejaculate just like a full bladder increases the urge to urinate.

That same idea might apply to the Skene's glands so that when they become more proliferative and fill with fluid, you might have increased libido and maybe even ejaculate and that's indeed what we've seen women start to ejaculate for the first time or have more intense orgasms and increased libido. We think it's due to a combination of rejuvenation of that tissue, increased blood flow to the tissue, increased sensation to the tissue, general overall improvement in the health of the urethra which we know as erotic sensations as well, and overall improved health of the mucosa of the vagina.

All these things are rejuvenated by the platelet rich plasma injected into this area. We've not done biopsy studies... we just have clinical reports of women's response to this. As of now, we have over 90% of women injected have improvement of their sexuality that's very easily measured and over 90% of them have resolution of their stress incontinence if they did not have a significant structural abnormality with their bladders coming out into their vagina or if they have rectocele where their rectum is coming through the wall of the vagina. That's a different problem but if they just have simple urinary incontinence, we have over 90% cure rate with this injection.

That's how the shot works. Let's talk more about some of the results and we'll cover more details of the science as we talk about more women who experienced the shot and how they've responded to it.

Chapter 4: The Second O-Shot® Ever-Anywhere

After the first O-Shot ®, when I saw how dramatically she responded to platelet rich plasma, I became hopeful that it might help someone who has difficulty with orgasm or sexual function. So, I called a friend whom I knew had severe pain with intercourse. We'll call her Theresa.

A Beautiful Banker's Secret

April 2011, I called Theresa and said, "I want you to come see me at lunch. Just come over on your lunch hour from the bank. I don't know if this will help you but I know the material I'm using won't hurt you. It's from your bloodstream and I can explain it to you when you get here but we need to try this."

She knew me and trusted me, so that's all the explanation she needed.

Theresa worked then at a bank a couple of blocks from my office. In her late 30's, a master's degree, smart lady, single mother with a son at 6 year's old.

She had divorced her son's father because of physical abuse including physical abuse of her genitalia to the point that she had scarring and pain with intercourse. She was *enduring* a relationship with a man that she didn't enjoy partly because of painful sex.

When she arrived at my office, she almost whispered to me, "Charles, I really don't like the man I'm with, but since I can't enjoy sex, I don't really feel like I can go out and find someone better."

Imagine being beautiful and loving but knowing that you have significant pain with intercourse so severe that whomever you're with is going to have difficulty having intercourse with you unless you use numbing cream—also making it impossible to experience pleasure. That was her situation.

That idea combined with her struggle to recover from an abusive relationship kept her trapped in solitude.

Theresa smiled and went on, "Before I was married, I was a sex addict. I loved sex! Loved orgasms, multiple orgasms, and often even ejaculated."

I put some numbing cream on tissue and said, "I hope I can help you. I don't know it this will work, but it might. Here. I'm going to leave the room and you put this numbing cream inside your vagina and on your clitoris."

I put a dot of cream on her arm where I would be drawing blood; then I left the room.

When I came back, I drew her blood, centrifuged it, and then injected it in the same way you've already heard me describe.

Theresa looked grateful but worried as she put on her dress to go back to work. She then gave me a big hug and I watched her walk down the stairs from my office to head back to the bank.

Later, that night around 9 PM, she texted me, "This is insane! I just had to pull my car off the side of the road to masturbate!!"

"Theresa," I texted. I'm glad things are better but this could just be the initial pressure from the injection. Only after 2 or 3 weeks will we know if the new tissue actually rejuvenated to the point of curing your dyspareunia."

A few hours does not allow enough time for stem cells to actually rejuvenate. But even though tissue growth becomes significant on the second or third week, in some women the initial response gives so much pleasure it becomes the ultimate "sex drug"—it gives extreme pleasure with the side effect of making you healthier!

3 weeks later, almost to the day, Theresa called to tell me that her pain was gone.

The next week, Theresa called to tell me how much better she was sleeping because she didn't have to get up in the night 3 or 4 times to urinate.

I remember how happy she sounded when she said, "Charles, that shot changed my life! I've lost weight and not depressed because I can sleep and exercise. Also, I think having the orgasms even with my vibrator makes me less anxious and depressed. I'm a better mother and I'm doing better at the bank just because I feel so much better."

So, she reported her urinary incontinence was gone so she was sleeping through the night and went back to jogging and walking daily. Her depression and anxiety went away. And she could have comfortable sex, all from a shot that took 15 minutes on her lunch hour!

About this time, she dumped the boyfriend.

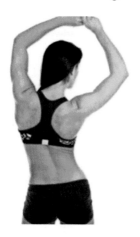

From O-Shot® to Wedding Bells

Two months later, she called me to tell me that she was now engaged to a man she had loved since high school, but they had not been seeing each other. Now, with her newfound health and sexuality and confidence, she called him. They rekindled their relationship and he asked her to marry him.

They married a few months after that and she continues to enjoy a healthy sexuality and no more urinary incontinence—and all this became possible because of a painless, near risk free, procedure that took 15 minutes on her lunch hour!

About 15 months after the first shot, Theresa volunteered to be a model in one of the courses I teach at my office to show the physicians how to do the O-Shot ® procedure. She came and told her story and we repeated the shot. Her sexual function was still doing very well and her dyspareunia was still gone. Her urinary incontinence was still gone but she said she was starting to dribble just a little.

So, we repeated the shot.

Once Is Magic—*Twice* is Ecstasy

After the second shot, as happens with many women, her sexuality went to levels higher than after the first shot. Her orgasms became much more intense. She started to ejaculate routinely. Not with every encounter, but more frequently with more intense orgasms and of course her urinary incontinence completely went away again. So she's had 2 shots now in about a little over 2 years and still doing very well.

A couple of things to learn from this are that, as was stated in the Journal of American Medical Association in 2009, Theresa demonstrates that sexual dysfunction is very distressing and can cause a whole change in a person's life. Because of the pain with her sexuality, it was affecting who she was spending time with... it was affecting her whole family. As in now her son has a new stepdad, there's a new loving model of loving relationship at home. She's happier and I think she's a better mother because of her happiness and less depression. She's lost now about 15 pounds and is healthier because she's running again and all of this from a shot with almost no risk that took her about 30 minutes total on her lunch hour.

Hopefully this gets to have another idea about how the shot might be helpful in rejuvenating and activating the Female Orgasm System.

You Can*NOT* Cure Everything with a Shot

I do not pretend that the shot somehow erases the psychological scars of abuse. Theresa was smart enough to have seen a counselor before the O-Shot ® procedure.

I do not think this shot is some magic thing that makes all hormones normal or heals all broken hearts. I don't want to make this into something more than it is. But, if someone goes to the best counseling and they have the best hormones but they still have vaginal tissue that's not healthy, it's like learning to be a racing car driver but having a car with a broken engine so it can't really get around the track very well. I think it's helpful to have a car that works and know how to drive it and shift the gears.

Theresa, as the second O-Shot ® procedure patient, taught me that the O-Shot® cures urinary incontinence. Let's talk about the science of how that happens in the next chapter.

Chapter 5: Urinary Incontinence

After treating Theresa with the O-Shot ®, I felt honored and amazed at how her life improved from just stopping her urinary incontinence: better sleep, the ability to exercise without embarrassment, and her depression gone because she could sleep and exercise. After seeing her results, I became more interested in how the procedure may benefit other women with urinary incontinence.

How to Know if Leaking Urine is Urinary Incontinence

First, consider the definition of incontinence. If you ask, "Do you ever drip a drop of urine into your underwear?"

Most men and women will answer, "Yes."

The International Continence Society formally defines urinary incontinence as the "Involuntary loss of urine that is either a social or a hygiene problem and is objectively demonstrable." In other words, when leaking urine either embarrasses you or causes problems with hygiene—then you've got urinary incontinence.

The risk factors for developing urinary incontinence at some time in your life include just being a woman! Other risk factors include childbirth, persistent cough, aging, obesity or smoking.

One research project showed that if you look at women ages 20-29, about 5% of them have urinary incontinence severe enough to really bother them. 5% may not sound like much until you consider that 5% is the same as 1 in 20 women!

Of course, the percentage increases as women age.

Solving the incontinence problem seems pretty simple: trying to keep water in a container with a tube that's leaking. No complicated metabolic problems, no malignancy, incontinence is just a simple mechanical problem of holding water (urine) in a container (the bladder).

So, you might think curing urinary incontinence would be relatively simple compared to curing cancer or solving world hunger. So, why do so many women still suffer?

Take a look at the available treatments.

Ways to Treat Urinary Incontinence

First, doctors usually recommend "behavior management."

An example of behavior management: simply go to the bathroom frequently. An example would be when you were a child and your mother told to urinate before you got in the car so she could drive without stopping. Another example: just go to the rest room every hour or so. A time schedule such as this works fine if you are in an environment where you can easily go whenever you want on schedule, but this is not always possible.

For example, I had a patient who is a massage therapist who had to do 90 minute massages. Even though she would urinate prior to massage, she sometimes could not make it through the whole 90 minutes without breaking to go to the restroom, so she had to keep herself mildly dehydrated. After the O-Shot ®, that problem went away.

You can try to stay dehydrated but the benefits of drinking adequate amounts of good water are vast. Not only does water help one stay mentally clear, it helps digestion, appetite suppression, and is essential in the prevention of urinary tract infections. The idea that people stay semi-dehydrated as an effort to avoid urinating on themselves is not an ideal.

Weight loss can help but is a difficult solution and not that helpful for most people. Kegel exercises can improve the situation but again does not cure most people who suffer with urinary incontinence. Behavior therapies are safe and work for some but are not ideal for most women.

Pills that Treat Incontinence

The next step up is medicines called anticholinergics. They can be very helpful and will continue to be available, but they have side effects. They can interfere with the ability to think, they can cause constipation, and they can make one feel dehydrated. For an older woman who may already have difficulty with memory, taking anticholinergic medicines to help with incontinence can tip her into a dementia that makes her unable to live alone. For a younger woman, urinary incontinence can bring a stop to cheerleading or gymnastics or other physical activities. If she takes anticholinergic medicine, it could interfere with her ability to work or to study. Anticholinergic medicines have their place but should only be used when appropriate and when tolerated; however, the side effects of these medicines make them unacceptable for many.

Surgery that Treats Incontinence

The next steps up from medicine are slings and meshes, which are needed for some people. If a woman's bladder is hanging outside of the vagina 2 inches into the womb, she needs a surgical procedure to hold that in place. Yes, there are people who have complications like erosions and infections but complications are rare. Surgery should be used when needed.

A sling can stop incontinence, but it can also cause obstruction as well as infection. It is a surgery that can cause scaring; therefore, it is not ideal (especially for a younger woman who intends to have children). It is a procedure that can be done and it will continue to be done even with the O-Shot®. It's a pretty invasive thing to do, a mesh or a sling. It's a pretty far step up compared to the behavioral therapies of just going to the bathroom frequently.

Injections to Cure Incontinence

The next step up from the anticholinergic medicines are injectables like Coaptite, which is a type of calcium hydroxyapatite crystal that can cause granulomas that must be surgically removed. These medicines do help some women with incontinence by causing a discreet constrictor, not an overall rejuvenation. Nearly half of the people who have the procedure done can have urinary obstruction, where they have trouble getting the urine out. Other problems that can occur are staff infections, bleeding and almost 1 in 20 is not cured by the procedure. And lastly it is painful.

Why Your Doctor Should Learn the O-Shot ® Procedure

Where I think the O-Shot ® comes into play is for those people for whom a time schedule or weight loss has not cured their urinary incontinence, and they're not suffering to the point to where they want to risk the side effects of taking the drugs previously mentioned.

The O-Shot ® can be placed and has the effect of rejuvenating the entire surrounding area of the urethra with over 90% having their urinary incontinence cured with 1 procedure. It seems to last somewhere around 1 to 2 years.

Even with the artificial injectable materials that are used to treat incontinence, there's a 41% incidence of urinary retention where the woman is not able to empty her bladder after the procedure. We have seen none, not one case, of that happen with the O-Shot ®. There can be see mild pain with the injection, but most report no pain. There are a few people who have dysuria, mild pain with urination for a day or two, and maybe even some mild spotting. It is an injection, so if I give you an injection in the shoulder, you'll have a spot or two of blood. The same thing can happen with this procedure, but there is no significant bleeding. In fact, the needle used is so thin, you could put it in your carotid artery and not bleed significantly.

Hopefully we'll see many people who are bothered and would have progressed to have a sling or a mesh not have to do those things because the O-Shot ® works for incontinence. However, even though it does indeed work well, it will not make other therapies go away, rather it is simply another tool to fill in the gap of incontinence treatment. There will continue to be people who need to have surgery.

It is important to understand that the number one reason for going into the nursing home is not dementia. People will continue to care for their mother at home when she becomes forgetful. It's not weakness. It's not inability to bathe. The number one reason for sending "Mother" to the nursing home is when she gets to where she urinates on the floor. Becoming too weak to hold urine is a significant problem. sit is then that the family gives up and says, "Now, I must send my wife or mother to the nursing home because I'm not able to take care of her."

Incontinence causes social problems in other ways. Incontinence was a nuisance for my 36-year-old friend who worked at a bank, making it difficult for her to sleep, but for an 80-year-old woman, incontinence   can   mean stumbling and breaking a hip in the night, it can mean urinating on the bed and having skin breakdown, it can mean even worsening of fatigue and trouble with thinking because of the interruption of sleep. Urinary incontinence is not the most horrible thing in the planet, but it is very horrible for those who suffer with it. We're seeing very good results. Over 90% of those who have the O-Shot ® see their urinary incontinence go away.

For those who would like to try the procedure for help with their urinary incontinence, providers are listed at oshot.info.

Chapter 6: Confessions of O-Shot ® Recipients

Most of the women who come for the O-Shot® or the male version (the Priapus Shot®) come because they value their love relationship. Either they're trying to start a new relationship, or they're trying to salvage a mature relationship that's damaged or stale. In other words, most who visit me or other providers for this do so because of love.

Single women enjoy sexual energy as well, and they seek out the O-Shot® as a way to heighten or enhance their sexual energy. As a result they find they have more mental energy, they feel more creative, they can connect more spiritually.

Some women already enjoy the benefits of excellent sex. They want superior health and want superior sexual health. The O-Shot® takes them to a whole new level of sexual experience.

Comments I've heard most often include the following: "rediscover each other's bodies," "we're closer than ever," and "we're like teenagers." To understand those comments, here are just a few samplings of hundreds of stories from some of the lives changed by the O-Shot® procedure.

Speed-Bump Orgasm

After doing the procedure for a few months, the results were so amazing that I decided I should teach other doctors to do the procedure and gather data. One of the first physicians for whom I showed the procedure practiced in Southern California.

First, I sent pictures and diagrams to show the doctor how to do the procedure but he and his partner did not see the same results as I had seen. So, I flew out to demonstrate the procedure. After arrival, I saw they were injecting the material the way they had been taught to inject man-made materials (like Coaptite®) and the location was not as effective as what I was doing. It was a simple correction, and they now see great results.

The first lady I treated when I went to their office was a friend of the doctor's. She came to the office, we drew the blood, we spun it in the centrifuge, and gave the injection. The next day was a Saturday. I came back to his office to watch him do more procedures and to give him feedback. Between patients, his cell phone rang.

It was the answering service. As he sat at his desk, I watched a worried look cover his face. Then he looked at me and said, "Charles, you should hear this," and handed me the phone.

It was the lady from the evening before and she was crying. She said, "I'm here alone and I've been masturbating all morning with anything I can find. I had the first orgasm when I hit the speed bump leaving the parking lot last night and now I can't stop masturbating! I'm so aroused that I want to go down the street to my neighbor's husband because I know she's gone and I do not even like the man. What do I do?"

What do you do with that?

This hypersexual response only happens in about 5-15% of the people who get the shot. When it happens, it's from pressure from the injected fluid, not because of the long lasting effects of the shot (which come from development of the stem cells into new and healthier tissue). Most see no benefit from the procedure until 2-3 weeks after the shot. It takes that time for the stem cells to regenerate new tissue to the point where the woman notices improvement. Maximal effect is in 3 months.

The extreme sex drive and orgasmic response seen in the first week could be a result of growth factors released from the platelets causing enhanced blood flow. More research will hopefully reveal the answer.

Still, lack of total understanding does not change the fact that for some women who are functioning well before the procedure, the O-Shot® can be like a recreational drug with women wanting to have the shot every time they go on a vacation or have a special date because they know it's not harming them, it's painless, and they experience intense pleasure for a week following the injection.

I wanted you to know that story so you know about the hypersexual response in case it happens to you. But, please realize that with around 95% of women, the results are more gradual.

Ejaculation Surprise

Soon after a New Orleans physician started offering the O-Shot® procedure, she received a phone call from Mary, a 65-year-old woman, who said, "That shot made me urinate on myself!"

So, the physician called me, very troubled. "What happened? I didn't know the procedure could *cause* incontinence. The patient came to improve her orgasms—which she did—but now she's incontinent."

I was puzzled. Over the phone, I said, "I didn't know it could do that either. I don't see how that could happen since the procedure rejuvenates tissue. After you talk with Mary in person and examine her, please call me and tell me what you find."

The next day, Mary visited the doctor. She told her doctor that during intercourse, she had the most powerful orgasm of her life during which she "urinated." That was the only time she had "lost her urine."

The doctor smiled and said, "Mary that was not urination. That was ejaculation."

Ejaculatory orgasms and strong, multiple orgasms can occur starting 3-4 weeks after the O-Shot® procedure. I wanted you to hear this story, so if that happens you won't be worried.

Big Baby Causes Big Problem

Two years ago, Susan (name changed), a 21-year-old woman who works near my office, delivered a 10-pound baby boy. Afterwards, Susan started suffering with pain every time she had sex with her husband—whom she loves deeply. She also developed difficulty holding her urine, which slowed her at work

Her gynecologist was not able to help her.

When Susan discovered the O-Shot® on-line, she volunteered to be a model for the procedure in one of the workshops I teach for physicians and nurse practitioners.

On the day of the workshop, Susan walked into the room and sat down on the couch to tell her story to the physicians there for instruction. She is very beautiful but very stoic. If you see her at work, she shows little emotion. But, within moments of starting to tell her story, her shield fell and she began sobbing.

Through tears she explained, "Since having my baby, I can't have sex with my husband because of the pain. We are almost through with the paper work—I'll be divorced in a couple of weeks. A huge part of our problem is that I can't have sex."

An article in the Journal of the American Medical Association from 2009 demonstrated that sexual dysfunction is more common in young women than in older women and that the psychological distress from sexual dysfunction is worse in women than in men. As I watched Susan sobbing, it was easy to feel her pain and how she may feel abandoned and unlovable and why that research could be true.

Regardless of how you believe Susan and her husband should have handled her problem, and regardless of what the full picture at her house might reveal; the fact remained that Susan's inability to experience pleasure with sexual relations put a severe strain on her marriage. In addition, this strain was contributing to a separation that would result in heartache and in a father visiting his child on the weekends rather than being present for nightly bed-time stories.

Susan also suffered with urinary incontinence that interfered with her work, but for her, incontinence was a minor nuisance compared with her marital problems.

I gave Susan the O-Shot® procedure for free for gifting the physicians with her story (it is a gift when people share their pain). Three weeks later, she texted me, "It feels like I woke up down there! No more pain!! □ □ The divorce is final now but we're back to having sex again!!"

Who knows if their relationship will heal, but she is once again enjoying sex and romance with the father of her daughter, which is certainly a step in the right direction. As a result of this procedure, she feels healed and whole as a person, and that restored feeling of well being will enrich all of her relationships.

Imagine being 21 years old, feeling damaged, unable to experience sexual pleasure with your husband and feeling inadequate to look for another relationship. Then imagine being restored with a painless procedure with almost no risk that took only a few minutes in the office. She called and said, "I want to be on standby if you ever need a model for another class, and I want all doctors to know about this procedure."

A couple of months later, I did need another model for another physician who came in for instruction. Susan took a 30 minute break from work and (because I already knew her medical history) just walked over had the treatment and walked back to her office—all during 30 minute break at work. So, though the physician doing the procedure the first time must understand the patient's medical history and physical exam, the procedure can be done with out much time or drama.

Also, after the second shot, as with many women, Susan saw the enhancement of her sexuality escalated to even higher levels: orgasms became explosive and tremendous and came more easily. And, her libido became even stronger.

Warning!

The O-Shot® procedure is a specific method of injecting PRP to rejuvenate the tissue of the vagina that is protected by US Patent & Trademark law. You'll find the procedure listed at www.uspto.gov by searching trademarks.

The trademark identifies physicians who meet the required standards and so may legally use either "O-Shot" or "Orgasm Shot" to advertise. Therefore, a woman who sees the "O-Shot" name knows the provider studied and agreed to the methods of the procedure. This does not promise a perfect outcome (no doctor can promise that), but it does promise the woman an excellent standard of care.

Many spin offs have and will occur where others claim better ways. Please beware.

Mapping is Not Needed

Some physicians may say they need to "map the vagina" and find the part of the vagina most sensitive. *In other words, they intend to sexually stimulate the woman's vagina in the office* to find the part of the vagina where the shot should be placed. This method of "mapping" was needed with previous procedures because the substance being injected did not spread--it was granular in nature. But, PRP spreads like water when injected. Because the area in question is so small and the amount of PRP injected is relatively large, the PRP will cover the entire area in question without mapping. Of course, the doctor must understand PRP and know where to place it in the vagina so it spreads properly. Anyone who claims that mapping of the vagina is needed for this procedure is not aware of this advanced technology known by the true O-Shot® providers.

"Mapping" only adds an extra degree of uncomfortable embarrassment for the woman for no legitimate scientific reason.

If your doctor says he needs to do "vaginal mapping"—run.

Good Doctoring Requires the Whole Picture

Please always remember that sexual response involves much more than just the vagina (as you now know from reading about the Orgasm System). Your doctor should talk to you about your physical and psychological health and be interested in blood testing of your hormones. If your doctor does not ask about those topics and offer ways (or a referral) to test and evaluate your overall health, find another   provider.

Physicians listed at www.OShot.info should be collecting data about your overall health, and they should NOT do vaginal mapping. There may be other spin-offs that are questionable. If you find a provider who seems questionable, or who advertises the O-Shot® or Orgasm Shot® but who is not listed at http://www.OShot.info, (no matter how many books or TV shows they've done) then please send an email to this address to let me know so that I can protect women who may be tricked: mailto:DrRunels@Runels.com

Nothing Perfect

Hopefully the stories in this chapter help you understand more about the procedure—how it works and what can happen. Of course, there is no perfect procedure, but I have seen, as well as the other doctors listed at www.OShot.info seen women who had the procedure and did not find relief.

Also, some simply are not candidates. If a woman suffers with the psychological effects of abuse, then this procedure will not heal those psychological wounds. If the woman has a "dropped bladder" or extreme pelvic floor weakness, then she may need a mesh or other surgical procedure.

A post menopausal woman not taking any hormones will be more likely to not see results from the procedure than a premenopausal or hormonally replaced woman. But, some post-menopausal women not taking hormones do experience the return of a strong sex drive and orgasm ability after the shot.

Some who seem to be hormonally replaced still don't respond to the O-Shot® procedure. But that happens in less than 2%. Most people, if they are hormonally replaced or pre-menopausal, if they have this procedure done, their sex and urinary continence will improve.

Now that you've learned more about the female orgasm system and the O-Shot® procedure, you will see improvements in your life. As you read the next chapter, I invite you to do something new to create something new in your life.

Chapter 7: Recipes for Sexual Healing

Remember if you want something new to happen, you must do something new. So, this is THE most important chapter in this book.

Do nothing new, and I can almost guarantee nothing will change. But, if you follow the plans below, I can almost guarantee that your life will improve.

Important: I'm writing what I've seen work best after taking care of thousands of women and doing clinical trials for the past 20 years. But, every woman is different and the only person who knows exactly what you need is your physician. So, trust your physician more than you trust this book.

On the other hand, if you've been seeing your physician for more than 6 months and your condition has not improved, then consider giving this book to your physician.

Some people will get three bids and spend a month interviewing people before getting their house painted but will jump at the first recommended physician and stick with them even if not getting better. You need to stay with the same physician long enough for her to learn your history and for you to try her strategies. But, if after 6 months you are not better, then that's a good sign that you should seek a second opinion. If I have a patient who's not improving, I always welcome the chance for another physician to take a careful look. None of us knows everything, and the best always welcome help.

Treatment Plans
(only with approval of your physician)

Find the Best Physician for You

- Ask the ***Guiding Question*** of your physician (or potential physician) to know if you're with the right person: "Would you consider adjusting my hormone levels (even if my levels measure in the "normal" range by blood testing) if I show signs and symptoms of disease; or, do you consider a "normal" blood test (even if low-normal) to be the overriding factor to guide your therapy?'

- Many of the physicians listed at www.OShot.info offer expert evaluation and treatment of the entire woman (not just expert with the O-Shot ® procedure.)

- Your physician may be a family practitioner, a gynecologist, an internist, or a nurse practitioner from one of those specialties. At the time of this writing, however, most endocrinologists of the USA tend to be behind the present thinking of the rest of the world.

- **When you find a doctor who answers "yes" to the Guiding Question, then use that doctor as your final authority (not this book) on what you should do for the following problems. Nothing substitutes for a physician who actually knows you and can do a physical exam.**

Pain with Sex (Dyspareunia)

- Check an ultrasound for pathology of ovaries or uterus. If ovarian cysts or uterine fibroids, these should be treated either medically or surgically.

- Take at least a week with no sex at all other than kissing and cuddling. This holiday can be extended up to a month. Enjoy activities other than vaginal stimulation with your lover.

- Exam and treatment of any infection or skin problems.

- Lubricants (KY Jelly still works).

- Estrogen and testosterone creams applied to the vaginal mucosa every night work well to help rejuvenate tissue.

- Vibrators of gradually increasing size. Start very small. Think of it as massage therapy and use the vibrator every night without expectations or attempts to achieve either stimulation or orgasm. Then, every week, increase the size of the vibrator (using a slightly larger size each week) until reach the size of your lover's penis if your lover is a man. Suggested vibrators can be found at www.FemaleOrgasmSystem.com.

- Rest from penis-in-vagina sex until comfortable with the vibrator. The woman will feel nervous and on guard until she can comfortably masturbate with a vibrator of the same size as her lover.

- Visit a reputable sex educator (suggestions on www.OShot.info/educators).

- Experience the results of the O-Shot ® procedure. Go here to find a certified provider: www.OShot.info. **Full effect of the shot takes 3 months. If desired effects not achieved after 10-12 weeks, repeat the injection.** May be repeated every 10 weeks until desired result obtained.

- Growing healthier vaginal tissue and changing brain chemistry/neurotransmitter levels takes time. This recipe takes 3 weeks before most women see any improvement. Full effect takes 3 months. After 2 months, repeat blood levels and consider adjusting dosages.

Decreased Sex Drive (Low Libido)

- Take at least a week with no sex at all other than kissing and cuddling. This holiday can be extended up to a month. Enjoy activities other than vaginal stimulation with your lover.

- Check and replace hormones. Free thyroid and free testosterone levels should be in the upper 25% of normal for a 30-year-old woman. I prefer blood testing. Estrogen and progesterone play less of a role for libido than does testosterone. I prefer testosterone injections or pellets (instead of testosterone creams) since absorption of the creams can be unreliable. Creams work very well to restore the vaginal mucosa and to help with pain because of strong local effects. But, they are not optimal for overall replacement for the entire body.

- If you're taking birth control pills (BCPs), consider using a different form of birth control. BCPs lower testosterone levels. If you choose to continue taking BCPs, then test blood levels of testosterone and supplement with testosterone if free testosterone is less than the upper 25% of normal.

- Experience the results of the O-Shot ® procedure. Go here to find a certified provider: www.OShot.info. Full effect of the shot takes 3 months. If desired effects not achieved after 10 weeks, repeat the injection. May be repeated every 10 weeks until desired result obtained.

- Growing healthier tissue and changing brain chemistry/neurotransmitter levels takes time. This recipe takes 3 weeks before most women see any improvement. Full effect takes 3 months. After 2 months, repeat blood levels and consider adjusting dosages.

Decreased Arousal

- Go here to find a certified provider of the O-Shot® procedure and make an appointment for evaluation and treatment: www.OShot.info. Full effect of the shot takes 3 months. If desired effects not achieved after 10-12 weeks, repeat the injection. May be repeated every 10 weeks until desired result obtained.

- Check and replace hormones. Free thyroid and free testosterone levels should be in the upper 25% of normal for a 30-year-old woman. I prefer blood testing. Estrogen and progesterone play less of a role for libido than does testosterone. I prefer testosterone injections or pellets (instead of testosterone creams) since absorption of the creams can be unreliable.

- If you're taking birth control pills (BCPs), consider using a different form of birth control. BCPs lower testosterone levels. If you do take BCPs, then test blood levels of testosterone and supplement with testosterone if free testosterone is less than the upper 25% of normal.

- Growing healthier tissue and changing brain chemistry/neurotransmitter levels takes time. This recipe hormonal recipe takes 3 weeks before most women see any improvement. Full effect takes 3 months. After 2 months, repeat blood levels and consider adjusting dosages.

Decreased Orgasm

- Experience the results of the O-Shot ® procedure. Go here to find a certified provider: www.OShot.info. Full effect of the shot takes 3 months. If desired effects not achieved after 10-12 weeks, repeat the injection. May be repeated every 10 weeks until desired result obtained.

- Check and replace hormones. Free thyroid and free testosterone levels should be in the upper 25% of normal for a 30-year-old woman. I prefer blood testing. Estrogen and progesterone play less of a role for libido than does testosterone. I prefer testosterone injections or pellets (instead of testosterone creams) since absorption of the creams can be unreliable.

- If you're taking birth control pills (BCPs), consider using a different form of birth control. BCPs lower testosterone levels. If you do take BCPs, then test blood levels of testosterone and supplement with testosterone if free testosterone is less than the upper 25% of normal.

- Consider oxytocin injections 30 minutes before sex.

- Go to www.FemaleOrgasmSystem.com and study free materials there.

Depression

- Work up to doing 21 miles of week of walking or jogging. Go here and listen to this recording to see how and why (best to do other activities but to not substitute other activities for the walking): www.drrunelsshow.libsyn.com/-1-weight-loss-health-   secret.

- Check and replace hormones. Free thyroid and free testosterone levels should be in the upper 25% of normal for a 30-year-old woman. I prefer blood testing. Estrogen and progesterone play less of a role for libido than does testosterone. I prefer testosterone injections or pellets (instead of testosterone creams) since absorption of the creams can be unreliable. Supplementing growth hormone levels can be very helpful as well; shoot for an IGF-1 level greater than 200. Prolactin levels if elevated will cause fatigue and depression and kill sex drive; make sure levels are checked and treated if elevated.

- If you're taking birth control pills (BCPs), consider using a different form of birth control. BCPs lower testosterone levels. If you do take BCPs, then test blood levels of testosterone and supplement with testosterone if free testosterone is less than the upper 25% of normal.

- Take SAMe 400mg on an empty stomach every morning. Wait 15 minutes before eating.

- Growing healthier tissue and changing brain chemistry/neurotransmitter levels takes time. This recipe takes 3 weeks before most women see any improvement. Full effect takes 3 months. After 2 months, repeat blood levels and consider adjusting dosages.

- Sit in a hot tub at 104 degrees F for 10 minutes followed by cooling off in a cool shower or cool pool.

- If you need to take an anti-depressant, request Wellbutrin (it can improve instead of hamper your sexuality).

Anxiety

- Work up to doing 21 miles of week of walking or jogging. Go here and listen to this recording to see how and why (best to do other activities but to not substitute other activities for the walking): www.drrunelsshow.libsyn.com/-1-weight-loss-health-secret.

- Check and replace hormones. Free thyroid and testosterone levels should be in the upper 25% of normal for a 30-year-old woman. I prefer blood testing. Estrogen and progesterone play less of a role for libido than does testosterone. I prefer testosterone injections or pellets (instead of testosterone creams) since absorption of the creams can be unreliable.

- If you're taking birth control pills (BCPs), consider using a different form of birth control. BCPs lower testosterone levels. If you do take BCPs, then test blood levels of testosterone and supplement with testosterone if free testosterone is less than the upper 25% of normal.

- Growing healthier tissue and changing brain chemistry/neurotransmitter levels takes time. This recipe takes 3 weeks before most women see any improvement. Full effect takes 3 months. After 2 months, repeat blood levels and consider adjusting dosages.

- Avoid alcohol. Using alcohol for anxiety leads to depression on top of the anxiety as well as weight gain and insomnia. If you drink alcohol, only do so when you are happy (not to treat depression or anxiety). Small amounts of alcohol can also make it MORE difficult for a woman to have an orgasm (even though it can decrease inhibitions).

- If you need to take an anti-anxiety drug, then that is what you need. You and your doctor decide. Just take as prescribed and do not use in combination with alcohol.

Fatigue

- Work up to doing 21 miles of week of walking or jogging. Go here and listen to this recording to see how and why (best to do other activities but to not substitute other activities for the walking):

- Check and replace hormones. Free thyroid and testosterone levels should be in the upper 25% of normal for a 30-year-old woman. I prefer blood testing. Estrogen and progesterone play less of a role for libido than does testosterone. I prefer testosterone injections or pellets (instead of testosterone creams) since absorption of the creams can be unreliable. Growth hormone levels can also be very important here; aim for an IGF-1 of greater than 200 (finding a physician in the US to prescribe can be very difficult).

- If you're taking birth control pills (BCPs), consider using a different form of birth control. BCPs lower testosterone levels. If you do take BCPs, then test blood levels of testosterone and supplement with testosterone if free testosterone is less than the upper 25% of normal.

- Growing healthier tissue and changing brain chemistry/neurotransmitter levels takes time. This recipe takes 3 weeks before most women see any improvement. Full effect takes 3 months. After 2 months, repeat blood levels and consider adjusting dosages.

Urinary Incontinence

- Start with physical measures: Kegels and frequent, scheduled trips to the bathroom. I'm not a fan of avoiding water as a way to treat since most people will enjoy better health (weight loss and better digestion and clarity of thinking) if they increase the amount of water they drink.

- Consult a certified physician to have an O-Shot® procedure. Whether your problem is stress or urge incontinence, this procedure is bringing much relief to women with almost no risk. Nothing works all the time for everyone, but this therapy has an over 90% chance of working unless you have major structural problems.

- PRP helps with healing of damaged tissue both immediately after an operation to improve healing and many years after operation to lessen scar tissue formation. So, if you've previously had a mesh or sling placed, you can still benefit greatly from an O-Shot ® procedure. you do have major structural problems and need a mesh or sling then that's what you need. You and your physician can make that determination. Even with all the bad-scary press, sometimes a mesh or sling is what's needed but be sure you try the O-Shot ® before you try the sling.

- If you do have major structural problems and need a mesh or sling then that's what you need. You and your physician can make that determination. Even with all the bad-scary press, sometimes a mesh or sling is what's needed but be sure you try the O-Shot ® before you try the sling.

Use the preceding lists only as suggestions. You and your physician should decide the best treatment for you. You can find physicians who understand the O-Shot ® procedure and who will work with your physician at http://www.OShot.info

References

1. Hom DB, Linzie BM, Huang TC. *The healing effects of autologous platelet gel onacute human skin wounds.* Arch Facial Plast Surg. 2007;9(3):174-183.

2. Sclafani AP, Romo TR III, Ukrainsky G, et al. *Modulation of wound response and*

soft tissue ingrowth in synthetic and allogeneic implants with platelet concentrate. Arch Facial Plast Surg. 2005;7(3):163-169.
3. O'Connell SM, Impeduglia T, Hessler K, Wang XJ, Carroll RJ, Dardik H. *Autologous* platelet-rich fibrin matrix as cell therapy in the healing of chronic lowerextremity ulcers. Wound Repair Regen. 2008;16(6):749-756.

4. Cervelli, Valerio MD; Lucarini, Lucilla MD.**Use of Platelet-Rich Plasma and Hyaluronic Acid in the Loss of Substance with Bone Exposure**. Advances in Skin & Wound Care: April 2011 – Volume 24 – Issue 4 – pp 176-181 *[This one shows using the same techniques used in the Vampire Facelift (R) procedure to grow new skin WHERE THERE IS NO SKIN]*

5. Redaelli, Alessio. *Face and neck revitalization with Platelet-rich plasma (PRP): clinical-outcome in a series of 23 consecutively treated patients.* Journal of Drugs in Dermatology – May 1, 2010

6. Azzena B, Mazzoleni F, Abatangelo G, Zavan B, Vindigni V. Autologous plateletrich *[Using Regen prepared platelet-derived growth factors (a single-spin centrifuge) to rejuvenate the face & neck]* plasma as an adipocyte in vivo delivery system: case report. Aesthetic Plast Surg. 2008;32(1):155-161.

7. Cervelli V, Gentile P, Grimaldi M. Regenerative surgery: use of fat grafting combined

with platelet-rich plasma for chronic lower-extremity ulcers. Aesthetic Plast Surg. 2009;33(3):340-345.

8. Cervelli V, Palla L, Pascali M, De Angelis B, Curcio BC, Gentile P. Autologous

platelet-rich plasma mixed with purified fat graft in aesthetic plastic surgery. Aesthetic Plast Surg. 2009;33(5):716-721.

9. Cervelli V, Gentile P. Use of cell fat mixed with platelet gel in progressive hemifacial atrophy. Aesthetic Plast Surg. 2009;33(1):22-27.

10. Cervelli V, Gentile P, Scioli MG, et al. *Application of platelet-rich plasma in plastic surgery: clinical and in vitro evaluation.* Tissue Eng Part C Methods. 2009; 15:1-9.

11. Sclafani AP. Platelet-rich fibrin matrix for improvement of deep nasolabial folds.J Cosmet Dermatol. 2010;9(1):66-71.

12. Sclafani AP. *Applications of platelet-rich fibrin matrix in facial plastic surgery.Facial Plast Surg.* 2009;25(4):270-276.

13. Sclafani AP. *Safety, efficacy, and utility of platelet-rich fibrin matrix in facial plastic surgery* [published online February 21, 2011]. Arch Facial Plast Surg. 2011;13(4):247-251.

14. Kakudo N, Minakata T, Mitsui T, Kushida S, Notodihardjo FZ, Kusumoto K.**Proliferation-promoting effect of platelet-rich plasma on human adiposederived stem cells and human dermal fibroblasts. Plast Reconstr Surg. 2008; 122(5):1352-1360.**

15. Oh DS, Cheon YW, Jeon YR, Lew DH. *Activated platelet-rich plasma improves fat graft survival in nude mice*: a pilot study. Dermatol Surg. 2011;37(5):619-625.

16. Danielsen P, Jørgensen B, Karlsmark T, Jorgensen LN, Agren MS. Effect of topical autologous platelet-rich fibrin versus no intervention on epithelialization of donor sites and meshed split-thickness skin autografts: a randomized clinical trial. Plast Reconstr Surg. 2008;122(5):1431-1440.

17. Anitua E, Sa´nchez M, Zalduendo MM, et al. Fibroblastic response to treatment with different preparations rich in growth factors. Cell Prolif. 2009;42(2):162-170.

18. Carroll RJ, Arnoczky SP, Graham S, O'Connell SM. Characterization of Autologous Growth Factors in Cascade Platelet-Rich Fibrin Matrix (PRFM). Edison, NJ:Musculoskeletal Transplant Foundation; 2005. Publication No. 128-XM 307C5.

19. Anthony P. Sclafani, MD; Steven A. McCormick, MD. Induction of Dermal Collagenesis, Angiogenesis,and Adipogenesis in Human Skin by Injection of Platelet-Rich Fibrin Matrix. Arch Facial Plast Surg.Published online October 17, 2011. *[Biopsy-proven new blood vessel growth and new collegen using platelet-derived growth factors (using a single-spin centrifuge)]*

20. Gafni-Kane, Adam MD; Sand, Peter K. MD. Foreign-Body Granuloma After Injection of Calcium Hydroxylapatite for Type III Stress Urinary Incontinence. Obstetrics & Gynecology: August 2011 – Volume 118 – Issue 2, Part 2 – pp 418-421doi:10.1097/AOG.0b013e3182161953 [showed a significant incidence of granuloma formation after injectin Radiesse like materials to treat urinary incontinence. Conclusion is that benefit is worth the risk].

21. Alijotas-Reig, Jaume MD, PhD. Foreign-Body Granuloma After Injection of Calcium Hydroxylapatite for Treating Urinary Incontinence. Obstetrics & Gynecology: November 2011-Volume 118- Issue 5-p 1181-1182 doi: 10.1097/AOG.0b-12e318235962d [Letter to editor challenging the idea that the benefit is worth the risk when using Radiesse like materials to treat stress incontinence--the point is that even with a risk of complications that require surgery, some gynecologist consider injecting around the urethera with Radiesse or Juvederm like material (i.e. the G-Shot™) to be an accepted practice. Yet with the PRP used in the O-Shot™ there seems to be ZERO risk of granuloma with even more benefit]

22. The American College of Obstetricians and Gynecologists,Practice Bulletin. Clinical Management Guidelines for Obstetrician-Gynecologists. No. 119. Apirl 2011 [Therapy available, hormones and psychotherapy--that's it]

About the Author

Charles Runels, MD did his undergraduate work and received his B.S. degree in chemistry from Birmingham-Southern College. He worked for three years as a product developer and researcher in physics & chemistry at Southern Research Institute designing instrumentation still used by the US armed forces.

He then completed medical school at the University of Alabama in Birmingham, after which he completed his residency and became board-certified in internal medicine.

During 12 years as an ER physician, he founded the largest group of ER physicians in his state while also serving as the medical director of a hyperbaric chamber used for wound care.

He then began a private internal medical practice and conducted clinical trials. He contributed to multiple, peer-reviewed, scientific publications in the areas of hypertension, hormone replacement, and immunology.

In cosmetic medicine, he designed and patented through the US Patent and Trademark Office specific ways of using growth factors to rejuvenate the face, commonly called the Vampire Facelift® and The Vampire Facial.

His professional organizations include the Association of Clinical Research Professionals. He founded the American Cosmetic Cellular Medicine Association (www.ACCMA.memberlodge.org) to help promote further investigation in that area.

His recent work includes research on urinary incontinence and sexual function in both men and women, resulting in his development of the O-Shot® (www.OShot.info) and the Priapus Shot® (www.PriapusShot.com).

He also works as the medical director for Accountability Health Care, supplying NP's and MD's to over 50 nursing homes in three states.

Based on his research, he coined the terms and developed the ideas of the "Female Orgasm System" and the "O-Spot" and authored books that include *Activate the Female Orgasm System* and *Anytime...for as Long as You Want: Strength, Genius, Libido, & Erection by Integrative Sex Transmutation* (which ran for three years as the best-selling sex manual on Amazon.com).

He is the father of three sons and lives in Fairhope, Alabama.

Charles Runels, MD
www.Runels.com

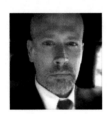

More Pathways to Better Sex

- *Discover if the O-Shot® procedure would work for you* or your lover. Tells physicians and nurse practitioners how to learn to do the procedure: www.OShot.info.

- *Find provider of the O-Shot®* procedure here: www.OShot.info/members/directory.

- www.OShot.info/books. Here you can find *books and other methods to help activate* the female orgasm system.

- www.OShot.info/educators. Gives location *of sex educators who understand* how to integrate the procedure into an overall plan for better sexual relations.

- www.FemaleOrgasmSystem.com. More details, including *free videos, about the female orgasm system.*

- www.PriapusShot.com. Method of using blood derived growth factors to *help sexual function in men.*

- www.VampireFacelift.com. Method for *rejuvenating the face* with blood-derived growth factors.

- www.OShot.info/physicians. Where physicians and nurse practitioners can apply to provide the procedure.

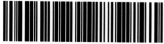

Made in the USA
San Bernardino, CA
08 November 2018